The Geographic Spread of Infectious Diseases

PRINCETON SERIES IN THEORETICAL AND COMPUTATIONAL BIOLOGY

Series Editor, Simon A. Levin

The Geographic Spread of Infectious Diseases: Models and Applications, by Lisa Sattenspiel with contributions from Alun Lloyd

Theories of Population Variation in Genes and Genomes, by Freddy Bugge Christiansen

Analysis of Evolutionary Processes, by Fabio Dercole and Sergio Rinaldi

Mathematics in Population Biology, by Horst R. Thieme

Individual-based Modeling and Ecology, by Volker Grimm and Steven F. Railsback

The Geographic Spread of Infectious Diseases

Models and Applications

Lisa Sattenspiel

with contributions from Alun Lloyd

PRINCETON UNIVERSITY PRESS

PRINCETON AND OXFORD

Published by Princeton University Press
41 William Street, Princeton, New Jersey 08540

In the United Kingdom: Princeton University Press
6 Oxford Street, Woodstock, Oxfordshire OX20 1TW

Library of Congress Cataloging-in-Publication Data

Sattenspiel, Lisa.
   The geographic spread of infectious diseases : models and applications
/ Lisa Sattenspiel with contributions from Alun Lloyd.
       p. cm. (Princeton series in theoretical and computational biology)
     Includes bibliographical references and index.
     ISBN 978-0-691-12132-1 (hardcover : alk. paper) 1. Communicable
diseases–Epidemiology–Mathematical models. I. Lloyd, Alun, 1970- II.
Title. III. Series.
     [DNLM: 1. Communicable Diseases–epidemiology. 2. Communicable
Diseases transmission. 3. Disease Outbreaks–statistics & numerical
data. 4. Epidemiologic Methods. 5. Models, Theoretical. WA 110
S253g 2009]
   RA643.S39 2009
   614.401'5118–dc22   2008038171

British Library Cataloging-in-Publication Data is available

This book has been composed in LATEX

The publisher would like to acknowledge the authors of this volume for
providing the camera-ready copy from which this book was printed.

Printed on acid-free paper. ∞

press.princeton.edu

Printed in the United States of America

10 9 8 7 6 5 4 3 2 1

Dedicated to Steven, Matthew, Elisabeth, and Stephanie who make my life a constant joy and to Franki and Ed (in spirit) who ultimately made this all possible. Love always — Lisa

The formidable task of developing models for endemic disease may be compared to building a house in a hurry. Practical workers insist on building a complete house, and are not too worried that it may need replacing later. Theoreticians insist on building reliable foundations and are not too worried if the house is never finished. Both points of view have their merits, and ideally we need to combine these.

— Mollison and Kuulasmaa, *Spatial Epidemic Models*

Contents

Preface

In early 2002, with the help of Alun Lloyd, Steven Tanner, Ben Bolker, and Tony Sun, I took on the task of creating a state-of-the-art review of models for the geographic spread of human infectious diseases, with particular attention to those models that were used for practical studies involving large epidemiological data sets. What was originally conceived of as a substantive review paper (50 pages or so) turned into a 250-page report. That report formed the nucleus for the present book, which has been updated and reorganized to reflect a recent astronomical rise in interest in modeling the geographic spread of infectious diseases. Credit for the core of chapters 2, 4, and 6 must go to Alun Lloyd; I mostly provided abundant critiques and revisions to supplement his clear exposition of the technical details related to modeling geographic spread. The majority of the rest of the book is primarily my work, although many of my ideas have been influenced by my numerous discussions with Alun about spatial modeling and its applications.

The goal of this book is to introduce how mathematical and computer models are used to study the geographic spread of infectious diseases. It is not intended to be a textbook from which one can learn all the relevant mathematical techniques and theory. Rather, it is designed to introduce the reader to the large body of work in this area, to stimulate discussion of the models and applications, and hopefully to generate enough interest in the field to draw new researchers to the area and help those already working in mathematical epidemiology to recognize new and interesting problems. The book is not intended to provide an in-depth analysis and review of all models that have been developed to study the geographic spread of infectious diseases. Rather, the focus is on those models that have been used in applications to actual epidemics, which means, of necessity, that many high-quality, but theoretically oriented studies are intentionally omitted from discussion.

The primary audience is readers who have background in ecology, epidemiology, human biology, and related natural, physical, and social sciences, and who have sufficient mathematical background to tackle the challenge of understanding the nature of model structures and basic analytical techniques. The mathematical level of the book is intended to be accessible to a wide audience that varies in mathematical skills, but the depth of discussion is such that advanced undergraduates, graduate students, and professionals in mathematics should still find much of interest, especially if they are relatively unfamiliar with epidemic modeling.

Numerous people contributed to the writing of this book. Alun Lloyd and I completed the bulk of the original report, but it benefited from the additional input of Steven Tanner, Ben Bolker, and Tony Sun, and that report would not have been possible without the financial support of the Defense Threat Reduction Agency. Innumerable colleagues have shared their work and/or commented on aspects of this project. I would especially like to thank the following people for their contributions: Cécile Viboud, Jorge Velasco-Hernandez, Richard Thomas, Pej Rohani, David Rogers, Mick Roberts, Les Real, Martina Morris, Denis Mollison, Martin Meltzer, Ira Longini, Simon Levin, Steve Leach, Uriel Kitron, Matt Keeling, Ed Kaplan, Mark Handcock, Peter Haggett, Bryan Grenfell, Rebecca Grais, John Glasser, Matt Ferrari, Steve Eubank, David Earn, Derek Cummings, Andrew Cliff, Carlos Castillo-Chavez, Tom Caraco, Donald Burke, John Bombardt, Chris Bauch, Frank Ball, Julien Arino, and Roy Anderson.

I thank Andy Dobson for his careful review of this manuscript and very helpful comments. The final version has benefited immensely from his critique. Connie Carpenter, Carolyn Orbann, and Karen Slonim carefully worked through the first three chapters of the book and provided abundant comments on the exposition. As graduate students in anthropology, they helped to ensure that the text met the goal of being understandable to a wide, not necessarily mathematically sophisticated audience.

Countless friends and colleagues, including the entire anthropology department at the University of Missouri, provided moral support and encouragement through the long process of bringing this project to fruition. Mary Porter, Gail Lawrence, and my family — Steven, Stephanie, Elisabeth, and Matthew — deserve special recognition. I couldn't have done it without them. Finally, I'd like to thank Sam Elworthy, my first editor at PUP, and Robert Kirk, Sam's replacement when he ran off to the other side of the world, who graciously put up with my relentless questions and stood by patiently until the project was completed.

The Geographic Spread of
Infectious Diseases

Chapter One

Introduction

In the fall and winter of 1918-19 a deadly epidemic of influenza, commonly known as the Spanish flu, erupted in Europe. Soldiers returning home at the end of World War I carried the epidemic to all parts of the world, eventually resulting in the death of at least 20-40 million people and perhaps significantly more (Crosby, 1989; Johnson and Mueller, 2002; Potter, 2001). The major epidemic was preceded by a short and less severe wave that occurred in the spring of 1918. This wave was similar in severity to other influenza epidemics and consequently was barely noticed by medical authorities (Crosby, 1989; Johnson and Mueller, 2002; Potter, 2001), although like the later, more serious wave, it was quickly carried throughout the world by soldiers and other travelers. It has also been suggested that outbreaks of an unusual influenza-like illness observed in England and France in 1916 and 1917 may actually have represented early outbreaks of the same flu strain as that which caused the major pandemic, and that these earlier outbreaks seeded the population of Europe and set the stage for the severe pandemic of the succeeding years (Oxford, 2001; Oxford et al., 2002). Furthermore, in at least some parts of the world the Spanish flu virus continued to circulate until at least 1920 (Johnson and Mueller, 2002).

In February 2003 the World Health Organization received reports of an outbreak of an unusual respiratory illness in China, with 305 cases reported and 5 deaths (Peiris et al., 2003). For the next 5 months, the world watched as this disease, given the name Severe Acute Respiratory Syndrome, or SARS, was carried throughout the world, eventually resulting in 774 reported deaths. From its start in China, the epidemic spread first to Hong Kong, then Vietnam, Singapore, Canada, and elsewhere, and although it eventually reached 26 countries on 5 continents, outbreaks with significant numbers of deaths were limited to only a few locations.

Both epidemics were caused by viruses that spread mainly through respiratory droplet transmission, both were carried rapidly across the globe, and yet the relative impact of the two epidemics differed markedly. What accounts for these differences? Were they due to dif-

ferences in the biology of the two viruses or in the biological response
of the human host? Or were they due to differences in the patterns
of social contact within and among populations? Was it a combination of both? Why did the Spanish flu kill tens of millions of people
while the SARS epidemic killed less than a thousand? What effects
did human responses have on the spread, morbidity, and mortality of
these epidemics?

A variety of approaches are being used to find answers to these
and other questions. Virologists have been called in to identify the
viruses that cause the diseases and determine whether specific biological features of the viruses influence their transmission and severity
of the disease process. It took a mere 6 weeks from the time the
World Health Organization received reports of the outbreak in China
until scientists successfully isolated the cause of SARS, a brand new
coronavirus (Peiris et al., 2003). The strain of the influenza virus responsible for the 1918-19 epidemic has been isolated from preserved
tissues of soldiers who died in the epidemic as well as from the tissues of at least one epidemic victim whose body was preserved in the
permafrost layer in Alaska (Taubenberger et al., 2000). Extensive
studies have been conducted to try to determine if the 1918 strain
possessed any unique biological characteristics that would explain its
unusual virulence, but, so far, a definitive answer continues to elude
researchers (Taubenberger and Morens, 2006a).

Table 1.1 compares these and other essential features of the 1918-
19 influenza epidemic and the 2003 SARS epidemic. A few biological
or epidemiological factors are clearly different for the two diseases,
especially the relative transmissibility (the ability to be transmitted
from one person to another), the importance of asymptomatic cases
in spreading the diseases, and the ages at highest risk for infection,
but the importance of these differences for explaining the observed
epidemic patterns has not yet been determined. Furthermore, although massive public health responses were mounted to try to stop
the spread of both diseases, the nature of the measures attempted and
the chances of their being successful differed significantly, given that
one epidemic occurred at the end of a long World War in the early
20th century while the other occurred at the beginning of the 21st
century at a time of relative world prosperity.

The 2003 SARS epidemic brought home the message to health authorities that many characteristics of modern society have increased
the risk that infectious disease epidemics will spread quickly across
time and space in the decades to come. Yet it is clear from looking
at the history of the 1918-19 flu epidemic that this is not really a

new phenomenon. In fact, our renewed interest in the 1918-19 epidemic has dramatically increased fears of new world-wide pandemics, precisely because the levels of travel present during the early 20th century were so much lower than now, and yet they were sufficient to spread a disease that resulted in the death of tens of millions of people. Although the SARS epidemic was not the world-wide pandemic that scientists feared, it still managed to spread to nearly every continent on Earth. This clearly points out how crucial it is to understand how, when, and why epidemics spread across the landscape so that effective planning, preparation, and control measures can be in place before a disaster occurs.

Humans have long recognized that travelers carry diseases from place to place. Setting limits on movement to control the geographic spread of diseases has been a common strategy since at least the time of the Black Plague epidemics in 14th-century Europe. In fact, the word quarantine is derived from the Italian words *quarantins* and *quarnta giorni*, which refer to a forty-day period during which ships, their goods, crew, and passengers were isolated in the Port of Venice during the 14th and 15th centuries (Markel, 1997). Italian authorities believed that an isolation period of 40 days would be sufficient to dissipate the causes of infections (Dorolle, 1968; Matinovic, 1969; Markel, 1997; Miller, 1993; Musto, 1988; Spencer, 1967).

Recognition of the importance of an activity in disease transmission does not guarantee that it will be addressed by scientists, however, and the spatial aspects of disease spread have more often than not been omitted from mathematical models, which have tended to stress who becomes infected, when they become infected, and why they become infected, but not where the transmission occurs and where the disease is spreading. Who, when, and why are important questions with answers that are necessary in order to determine how resources can be targeted to treat cases and institute preventive measures, but where the disease is predicted to spread is equally important.

The diffusion of a disease across a landscape is aided by the presence in space of a susceptible population and prevented by barriers of nonsusceptible persons or by empty space (Meade and Earickson, 2000). Geographic models can help us understand where a disease is likely to go given the local structure of barriers and susceptible populations, and can also help to determine where barriers should be placed in order to prevent further spread. For example, although the limited extent of the SARS epidemic is not fully understood, it is almost certain that kinship links and travel to visit relatives and friends on different continents provide at least a partial explanation of why

Table 1.1 A comparison of the influenza and SARS viruses

Feature	1918-19 flu	SARS
Observed characteristics:		
Epidemic length	multiple waves for at least 1 yr	single epidemic of 8 months duration
Cases	not known	8000+
Deaths	20-40 million	774
Geographic characteristics:		
Geographic distribution	world-wide	26 countries on 5 continents
Pattern of spread	variable depending on wave	China to Hong Kong to Vietnam, Singapore, Canada, elsewhere
Mechanism of spread	mostly rail, ship; troop movements	air travel
Mode of transmission, cause, and primary risk factors:		
Mode of transmission	respiratory droplets	respiratory droplets, fecal-oral?
Cause	new strain of known human virus	new human virus
Ages most affected	under 60; young adults especially hard hit	over 60
Specific risk factors	soldier; pregnant female	health care setting
Epidemiological parameters:		
Infectiousness	moderate	moderate
Transmissibility	moderate	relatively low, but possibly superspreaders
Estimated R_0*	1.5-2.5	2-4 early on; later 1.2-1.6
Incubation period	1-4 days	2-10 days; median 4-7 days, mean 6 days
Asymptomatic cases	significant	not important
Transmission before onset of symptoms	possible	not significant
Transmission after onset of symptoms	possible	possible
Global case fatality rate	variable; average 3%; up to 80% or more	about 10%

*R_0 is the average number of secondary cases caused by a single infectious person introduced into a population consisting only of susceptible persons

Canada was the only place outside Asia that experienced significant numbers of deaths from the disease. As noted in Gould (1989), "ignoring the spatial dimensions of [an] epidemic [is] like predicting the time of an eclipse, but being unable to tell people where they [can] see it."

The earliest work on the geography of disease centered on mapping, a practice that began as early as the 18th century (Cliff, 1995). By the middle of the 19th century maps of disease distributions were in widespread use and began to be used for hypothesis testing. Mapping is still the foundation of much work on infectious disease spread, and a number of new and complex statistical techniques have been developed to aid in this research. Nonetheless, although progress has been made with mapping techniques, other methods have been developed that provide better explanations for how and, more importantly, *why* infectious diseases spread across the landscape. Many of these methods have been drawn from disciplines other than geography, most notably ecology, epidemiology, and mathematics.

In this book we focus on one major area of study, mathematical epidemiology. Much of the work dealing with spatial aspects of infectious diseases traces its roots to the spread of animal and plant diseases and questions about the spatial distribution of resources. In large part, however, we have chosen to concentrate our discussion on the transmission and geographic spread of human infectious diseases and so we, of necessity, omit many studies that contribute to a wider understanding of the spatial spread of infectious diseases. Furthermore, although there is much theoretical work on this topic that has been of great value to the field of mathematical epidemiology, because of space limitations and personal interests our emphasis in this book is on applications of geographic models. Consequently, we focus on describing and evaluating the methods and results of models that have had their predictions tested by data, although promising approaches that have not yet been validated with existing data are still considered.

1.1 MATHEMATICAL MODELS AND THE GEOGRAPHIC SPREAD OF EPIDEMICS

Most disease models have been used historically to understand the naturally occurring introduction of known diseases and their subsequent spread within and, in some cases, across populations. This still is an important goal of disease modeling activities, but two situations in the modern world have brought epidemic modeling much more into the limelight. These situations include the emergence of new pathogens, such as SARS or the 1918-19 influenza, not seen before in human populations and the deliberate release of pathogens into human populations, or bioterrorism. By their very nature, the biology and epidemiology of new pathogens are not well understood. And epidemics due to the deliberate release of pathogens are likely to be fundamentally different from natural epidemics, for the simple reason that the pathogen release is likely to involve more than one source and be placed to maximize the rate of spread through a population.

Traditional statistical and mathematical analyses of data from past epidemics may not be suitable to deal with either of these situations, primarily because relevant data and knowledge on which to base the analyses do not exist. As this book will illustrate, mathematical modeling techniques are an important addition to the arsenal of epidemiological tools, especially since they can take advantage of the very limitations in data that compromise other techniques. Computers and computational strategies have become sophisticated enough to allow the development and analysis of more complex and realistic mathematical models. These models are based on an understanding of the fundamental biology of a host-pathogen interaction, and as long as a new disease is relatively similar to known diseases, models can be developed that reflect the underlying biology. In addition, known or suspected differences between the biology of previously known diseases and the new disease can be built into the structure of a model. The model can then be used to predict the outcome of an epidemic, even though humans may have had little prior experience with the disease. Although the predictions are likely to be imperfect, they provide some information with which to respond to the disease.

To take a recent example, mathematical models were used in the very early days of the SARS epidemic to help determine not only how serious the epidemic might become, but also to explore the potential impact of different proposed control measures (e.g., Chowell et al., 2003, 2004; Lipsitch et al., 2003; Riley et al., 2003). Insights from these models were used to show that the virus, if unchecked, could cause a significant epidemic, but that basic epidemiological control measures such as patient isolation and contact tracing could have a substantial impact on the extent of the epidemic. These activities on the part of public health authorities proved to play a major role in limiting the spread of the 2003 epidemic. The structure of the models was overly simplified, especially with regards to heterogeneities in contact and transmission, which were shown to be significant during the epidemic

(Dye and Gay, 2003), but, nonetheless, the models provided important guidance to public health authorities at a critical time when little other information was available.

So besides helping to predict and control the spread of new pathogens like SARS, what else can mathematical models do? They have a number of important uses. For instance, they can be used more generally to help elucidate important patterns in epidemiological data from any epidemic and can help us to further our understanding of the forces that generate these patterns. Sometimes the resulting insights may appear to be common sense in retrospect, but their significance may not be recognized until illustrated with a well-posed model. Mathematical models can also be used to help figure out how important different types of data may be for understanding and predicting disease spread and they can point out fundamental uncertainties in the existing data.

One of the most important roles of epidemic models is that they provide a way to experiment on human populations without actually doing invasive research that would be ethically unacceptable or technically unfeasible. For example, mathematical models can be used to help determine what might happen if a person was infected with deadly disease and then released from the hospital while still infectious to resume normal activities in a community. Essentially, mathematical models are best used as a way to enhance our basic understanding of how a complex system works. Furthermore, a model that is well-structured and adequately tested can be used to answer "what-if" questions about the behavior of a system that may aid in both the prediction of future behavior and the development of ways to alter that behavior, if desired. This process allows authorities to choose the control strategy most likely to be successful given existing, but often limited, knowledge and put it into place before an emergency occurs.

In a practical sense, a common goal of epidemic models is to aid in testing the feasibility of different control strategies at the community or larger scale. In order to do this, however, mathematical models must address a number of questions about the patterns of epidemic spread. A good model must be able to capture the most important details of the mechanism of spread both within a population and across the space that links different communities. However, a mathematical model is always a simplified description of reality. An important task facing a modeler, therefore, is to decide the level of detail at which the model will attempt to describe the system of interest. Although all models incorporate simplifying assumptions, a model that is too simple will not represent reality adequately, while a model that in-corporates too much of the detail in the real world will result in less general results that may not be applicable to situations other than the one being modeled.

There are no hard and fast rules about how much detail to incorpo-rate into a model, but there are a number of important considerations to keep in mind. The intended use of a model is probably the most important factor guiding model formulation. At the very beginning of the modeling process it is essential to know the questions one wants answered, because the structure of the model needs to be adequate to address those questions. For instance, if spatial dynamics are of interest then the model must contain some description of the spatial structure.

It is also essential to have a thorough understanding of the particu-lar biological system being modeled so that the model structure is an adequate representation of that system. Lack of detailed knowledge of a particular process, however, does not prevent its inclusion within a model, but this will necessitate making additional assumptions re-garding the process.

In a perfect world a modeler would have available any data needed to estimate the model parameters, but, unfortunately, data are almost always inadequate in real situations. Sometimes a modeler is in the position to collect the necessary data, but more often the availability of data dictates the modeling approach to be employed. In the ab-sence of good-quality epidemiological data, the benefit of generating highly detailed models is questionable, as the lack of data prohibits parameter estimation and model validation. When data are available, the behavior of the model can be compared to that seen in reality; differences in behavior may indicate deficiencies of the model, which require modifications to be made.

Often these modifications include the incorporation of additional biological processes within the model, with a corresponding increase in the number of variables needed to specify the state of the system and the number of parameters needed to specify the model. In some situations, such parameters can be estimated independently of the data set at hand. For instance, in an epidemiological setting, demo-graphic parameters can be estimated from population census data, without reference to data regarding the disease. If this is not the case, then the inclusion of additional parameters can be problematic because their values will have to be estimated using the disease data set.

Although statistical techniques can be used to provide these estimates, simultaneous estimation of several parameters can involve a complex optimization process, and general statistical theory shows that the more parameters that are to be estimated from a given finite data set, the less precise their estimates become. Care must also be taken to avoid overfitting a model to a given data set: the flexibility of a model increases as its number of parameters increases, and so it should not be surprising that a model with many parameters can fit a given data set better than a model with few parameters. In general, epidemic modelers should employ the practice known throughout science as Occam's razor, or the strategy of developing the simplest model that is consistent with observed behavior.

The reliability of models is another important consideration. Policymakers must have confidence in the recommendations that come from an epidemic model. This confidence can only come from comparisons of model predictions with data from actual epidemics — animal, plant, and human. At the very least a model should be able to explain some of the observed epidemic patterns, although it is important to realize that detailed geographic patterns of an epidemic cannot be replicated exactly, partly because of the inherently stochastic nature of real epidemics and partly because of a lack of adequate spatial data. For example, models of the geographic spread of rabies (e.g., Ball, 1985; Jeltsch et al., 1997; Murray et al., 1986; Murray, 1987), can reproduce the year by year wave advances of the disease measured in kilometers, but cannot predict where the disease will be in a more localized area. Recent advances in modeling techniques using hybrid models that combine dynamic models and statistical analyses have begun to more effectively model the actual heterogeneities present in real landscapes (e.g., Smith et al., 2002), but data of sufficient resolution to estimate needed model parameters are not yet available (Grenfell, 2002).

Mathematical models for the geographic spread of human infectious diseases require knowledge about detailed short-term mobility patterns of humans in the course of their daily activities, since those activities are directly responsible for disease spread across space. Human movement patterns are complicated and difficult to study, however. Data sets that would aid in understanding these patterns are probably available but scattered in various proprietary locations. For example, Baroyan and colleagues used airline and other transportation data to estimate mobility in their studies of the geographic spread of flu epidemics (cf. Baroyan et al., 1969, 1971; Baroyan and Rvachev, 1978; Rvachev and Longini, 1985), a strategy that has been used by several other investigators, including Aguirre and Gonzalez (1992),

Bonabeau et al. (1998), Flahault et al. (1988, 1994), and Freeman (2002). Eubank and colleagues have developed epidemic models that have at their core detailed data on the use of bus transportation in a western U.S. city (Eubank et al., 2004). Other potential sources of data on population travel patterns might include traffic counters along major roads or records from credit card use or hotel stays. The difficulty of acquiring and condensing such complex data into usable packets has led some researchers (e.g., Kaplan, 1989; Kaplan and Lee, 1990) to ask the question of whether detailed information about daily activities or complex social structures is truly necessary to understand observed patterns of disease, and, if so, exactly how detailed the data and the model using it need to be in order to adequately reflect the real situation.

Useful models must also be able to be generalized to different infectious diseases and geographical conditions or must be readily adaptable to specific conditions. As conditions change in the progress of the disease, the model must be able to be updated quickly to the new conditions. Of course, the results from the model must be available quickly so that they can be used before the real-time epidemic runs its course.

A particular strength of modeling approaches is that they can allow not only for generalizations to different infectious diseases, but also for generalizations across many different systems — epidemic modelers can often draw upon theory from other population biology settings. In particular, epidemiological systems can often be viewed as predator-prey processes, and so there are many direct analogies between ecological and epidemiological theory. The large body of work on ecological invasions is particularly informative with regard to the study of disease invasion. Conversely, many ecologists have shown interest in epidemiological systems because of the importance of disease in regulating the sizes of natural populations and because better data are often available for epidemiological systems than for ecological ones.

These crossovers among different areas of population biology are often reflected in the types of questions that are asked by modelers of disease processes. For example, epidemiologists are often most interested in practical questions related to epidemic prediction and control strategies. Hence, a modeler taking an epidemiological approach to developing models that take advantage of the large data sets on childhood diseases in Western Europe and North America may ask questions about when the next epidemic will occur, where it is likely to spread, and how effective different control strategies may prove in the face of an epidemic. Ecologists, on the other hand, are often more interested in understanding the underlying population dynamics and how they change over time, so an ecological modeler might use the same data set and a similarly structured mathematical model to answer how and why disease levels fluctuate within a community over long periods of time and whether such variation is due to random effects or nonlinear ("chaotic") dynamics.

1.2 STRUCTURE OF THIS BOOK

The remainder of this book will illustrate how mathematical models have been applied to understanding the geographic spread of recent and potential epidemics occurring in modern human and domesticated animal populations. Our goal is to provide content that will be accessible to a wide audience that includes both students and professionals in the biological, epidemiological, and social sciences as well as in mathematics. In-depth discussions of the structure and results of models that have been used to study and understand the patterns of spread of particular epidemics occurring in the recent past will be interspersed with discussions of the essential mathematical concepts and techniques used in these applications.

In Chapter 2 we introduce many of the important concepts used to motivate, structure, and analyze epidemic models in general before we delve into the additional complexity of models concerned with geographic spread. In the remaining chapters we alternate chapters dealing with applications of mathematical and computer models to the geographic spread of infectious diseases with chapters centered on issues related to model structures and analysis. Readers who carefully work through these chapters will be introduced to a number of modeling approaches as well as specific and extensive examples of their use within the literature.

Chapter Two

The Art of Epidemic Modeling: Concepts and Basic Structures

Mathematical models of the geographic spread of infectious diseases are, in almost all cases, adaptations and generalizations of models developed to explore disease transmission within a single population. Because the single-population models are much simpler in structure, and since many of the most useful results derived from epidemic models were first developed in the context of simple models, a general understanding of the important concepts is easier to grasp with single-population models. Consequently, in this chapter, we discuss the basic notions of model formulation for nonspatial models and the practical concepts and insights derived from them. These basic concepts will lay the foundation for understanding the structures and applications of spatial models in the following chapters.

The intent of this chapter is to describe fundamental epidemiological models, to discuss some of the most important issues related to epidemic modeling, and to develop just those concepts that are necessary to understand the discussion of later chapters. There are excellent texts that provide more complete introductions to epidemic modeling; see, for example, Anderson and May (1991), Brauer and Castillo-Chavez (2001), Diekmann and Heesterbeek (2000), Keeling and Rohani (2007), and Murray (1989).

2.1 ESSENTIAL BIOLOGICAL AND EPIDEMIOLOGICAL CONCEPTS

Epidemiological modeling usually begins with the development of a mathematical representation of an epidemiological process so that the behavior over time of this process can be studied. In order to do this effectively it is essential to have a firm understanding of the underlying biology of the system being modeled. By definition, epidemiology is the study of diseases in populations, but populations are made up of individuals, so most models of populations begin with assumptions about the disease process in the individuals that make up the population. These assumptions are made in relation to the biology of the specific disease being modeled, but many different kinds of infectious diseases share a fundamental structure that forms the basis for many epidemiological models. In this section, we describe some of the most important aspects of an infectious disease process within individuals and we provide a framework that is commonly used to represent this process during the development of an epidemiological model.[1] In the following section we use this framework to describe a simple epidemiological model that serves as the foundation for the majority of more complex models.

An individual who is considered to be at risk for infection with a particular pathogen is called *susceptible*. In order for that individual to move out of the susceptible stage, he or she must come into contact with an infectious stage of the pathogen. For some diseases this occurs through contact with an *infectious* individual who is infected with the pathogen *and* is capable of transmitting that pathogen to others. In other cases, the susceptible person must come into contact with another kind of infectious organism (e.g., a mosquito or rabid raccoon).

There are a number of different mechanisms by which pathogens make their way from one host to another — epidemiologists refer to these mechanisms as the mode of transmission. The most common modes of transmission are 1) respiratory, including droplet transmission, which occurs when infectious organisms are passed through the air from one person to another because of coughing, sneezing, talking, etc.; 2) fecal-oral, which can occur when pathogens in fecal material from an infectious individual are introduced orally to a susceptible individual; 3) sexual; 4) vertical or congenital — transmission from mother to infant, either *in utero* or during the birth process; 5) direct physical contact with infectious lesions; and 6) vector-borne — transmission that occurs indirectly when another living organism, most commonly a mosquito, flea, tick, or other arthropod, spreads the pathogen between host individuals. Many of these transmission modes will be illustrated in discussions of particular models or in applications chapters.

Once susceptible individuals become infected with a pathogen (also called the *onset of infection*), the disease progresses through a series

---

[1]Fine (2003) describes a similar framework and provides an excellent discussion of the different components of the framework, with particular emphasis on its practical epidemiological uses.

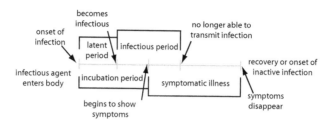

Figure 2.1 Progression of an infectious disease in an individual. See text for a more detailed description of each stage. Note that the infectious period may begin at or after the time symptoms appear and it may end at or after the time at which symptoms disappear.

of stages that are specific to the particular pathogen with which they have become infected. These stages are fairly well-defined for most pathogens, although in practice it can be difficult to determine precisely when particular stages begin and end. In addition, the length of each stage often varies not only between different pathogens but also among individuals who have been infected with the same pathogen.

Figure 2.1 illustrates the progression of an infection from the time an individual becomes infected until recovery or death occurs. At the onset of infection, for most diseases, a person enters both the *incubation period* and the *latent* (or *latency*) *period*. The incubation period is the length of time from the initial infection until a person develops symptoms of the infection and can be recognized by others as being infected; the latent period is the length of time between infection and the ability to infect another person, regardless of whether infection is apparent to others. The incubation period is often somewhat longer than the latent period, because the latter frequently ends before symptoms appear. This has important implications for the transmission and control of many pathogens, because transmission of the pathogen can and often does occur before anyone is aware of illness.

The end of the latent period signals the beginning of the *infectious period*, while the end of the incubation period signals the beginning of *symptomatic illness*. By definition, the infectious period lasts until the person can no longer transmit the pathogen, regardless of whether symptoms have disappeared or not. Often the infectious period is over before symptoms subside, but it is also possible for this period to end at the time symptoms disappear, and it is even possible for a person to remain infectious beyond the symptomatic period. For many but not all diseases, once the infectious period ends, a person enters a state of immunity to reinfection, which may be either temporary or permanent.

Death due to the pathogen may occur at any time during this process, although it most often occurs during symptomatic illness. The chance of death depends upon many factors, including not only characteristics of the disease itself, but also the underlying health of the infected individual, as well as contributing environmental factors such as quality of health care and sanitation levels.

In addition to these basic biological concepts, several epidemiological concepts are of importance in understanding the spread of epidemics. When a disease is present in a population at a relatively constant (usually low) level at all times, epidemiologists refer to it as an *endemic* disease; when the number of cases in a relatively localized area increases above the usual level for a short time the disease is said to be *epidemic*; when the disease reaches epidemic status within a short time span over large parts of the world, it is said to be *pandemic*.

Epidemiologists also use a pair of words to discuss the number of cases of disease: *prevalence* is used to refer to the total number of cases of a disease in a given population during a particular time interval, while *incidence* is used to refer to the number of *new* cases during a particular time interval. An epidemic or pandemic occurs when the incidence of a disease increases rapidly, whereas an endemic disease shows little or no change in incidence over time. High prevalence rates can be associated with pandemic, epidemic, or endemic situations, as can low prevalence rates. For example, an epidemic of a disease with low prevalence can come about if the normal prevalence rates are near zero but there is a brief and sudden rise in case numbers, as the last several years has shown to be the case with SARS. Similarly, an epidemic of malaria could occur after a boom in the mosquito population, even though the overall prevalence is high in endemic regions.

These biological and epidemiological concepts form the basic framework used to design the vast majority of epidemic models. In the rest of this chapter we shift our discussion to the process by which these ideas are translated into mathematics. In addition to describing in some detail the structure and analysis of a basic epidemiological model, we discuss basic modeling principles necessary to go beyond the simple models to those that are more complex and realistic.

2.2 THE CORNERSTONE OF MANY EPIDEMIC MODELS — THE SIR MODEL

To begin the process of developing an epidemic model, researchers generally begin with a disease progression scenario for a particular disease. In these scenarios it is convenient to classify individuals within the population according to their disease status; for example, susceptible (usually represented by S), exposed (E), infectious (I), or recovered (R).

The most frequently used foundation for more complex models is a simple model called the SIR model. This model includes two fundamental assumptions: 1) that a pathogen confers permanent immunity following recovery, and 2) that the latent period is so short that it can be ignored. Under these conditions the population being modeled can be divided into three groups on the basis of infection status: 1) susceptible (S) — individuals who are at risk of becoming infected, 2) infectious (I) — individuals who are capable of transmitting the pathogen to susceptible individuals, and 3) recovered or removed (R) — individuals who have recovered and so play no further part in the epidemic process. The name of the model arises from the three disease states (susceptible/infectious/recovered) included in it.

Sometimes the biology of a particular disease is such that the SIR model is not a good fit and so other similar formulations are used instead. For example, in some diseases, such as untreated gonorrhea, once individuals become infected they remain infected throughout their lives. Diseases like this would be modeled using only two stages, susceptible and infectious (SI models). Some diseases confer only temporary immunity, so models for these diseases would consider the progression from susceptible to infectious and recovered and back to susceptible (SIRS models). For many diseases the latent period is long enough that it cannot be ignored. This stage is usually modeled by including an exposed (E) stage prior to the infectious stage. As an example, models for diseases with latent periods and full immunity following recovery (e.g., measles) are usually designated as SEIR models.

The SIR, SI, SEIR, SIRS, and other similar models are examples of a type of model called a compartmental model (Jacquez, 1996). Compartmental models have wide applicability throughout the sciences. They are most often used to model a process by which some substance flows through a series of stages over time. For example, compartment models are used to describe such things as the flow of water through a series of tanks, to describe how a drug is distributed through different tissues in the body, or to model how cars are built as they move along an assembly line. Discrete individuals do not really exist in such models; rather it is assumed that individuals within the population, who may vary in their underlying characteristics, can be represented by a group of idealized individuals who are all identical to the population norm. In other words, variation among individuals is assumed to be unimportant (an assumption that is strictly valid only for large populations).

In compartment models it is assumed that the population can be specified solely in terms of the numbers of individuals of each type, who "reside" within particular compartments. At any given time a certain fraction of the population in one compartment flows into the next compartment, and this fraction need not be constrained to integer values. In the case of the SIR model, the population is specified in terms of the numbers of of susceptibles, infectious, and recovereds: S, I, and R. (Other notations can be found in the literature. For example, some authors denote the numbers of susceptibles, infectious, and recovereds by X, Y, and Z, respectively.) Each time unit a fraction of the susceptible subpopulation becomes infected and flows to the infectious compartment, and a fraction of the infectious subpopulation recovers and flows to the recovered compartment. This provides a population-level description of the system. For now, we restrict attention to a formulation of the model in which the movements of "individuals" between the compartments of the model are assumed to occur continuously.

The designation SIR is used for all models consisting of only the three compartments, susceptible, infectious, and recovered, but there are actually a number of models within that class, depending upon what other kinds of features are included. The simplest SIR model considers just two processes, infection and recovery, and both of these processes are assumed to occur at a constant rate. All other population processes (for example, births and deaths, or migration), are assumed not to occur.

Susceptible individuals can acquire infection by encountering infectious individuals. Contact between susceptible and infectious individuals is necessary for transmission, but it is not sufficient — the pathogen must also be transferred from the infectious individual to the susceptible individual, and that may not always occur. Consequently, the transmission rate can be thought of as a function of the average number of contacts, c, made by susceptible individuals and the probability p that a contact with an infectious individual actually results in transmission of the pathogen.

Many epidemic models assume that the overall transmission rate is the product of the two parameters c and p. In fact, in the simplest description of transmission the two factors, contact and probability of infection, are not explicitly recognized; rather, the infection rate is assumed to equal $\beta SI/N$, where β is constant. New infections arise at a rate that is proportional to the number of susceptibles and the probability that a given contact is with an infectious individual, I/N. The constant of proportionality, β, is known as the transmission parameter. (Remember, though, that this implicitly includes contact and the probability of infection given contact.) The per-susceptible rate at which new infections appear is called the force of infection, and some authors denote its value by the symbol λ, although this notation is not universal. For our simple SIR model the force of infection is given by $\lambda = \beta I/N$.

This depiction of the infection process generates the following equation for the transition from the susceptible to the infectious compartment:

$$\dot{S} = -\beta SI/N . \tag{2.1}$$

In this equation and throughout this book, a variable with a dot over it refers to the time derivative of the variable, i.e., $\dot{S} = dS/dt$.

Recovery leads to a flow from the infectious class to the removed class. The simplest description of recovery assumes that the rate of recovery is constant for each individual and equals γ, where the average duration of infectiousness is given by $1/\gamma$. (In other words, if infectious individuals recover at a rate of 20% per day, then the average duration of infection is $1/0.2$, or 5 days.) Assuming that individuals recover independently, the number of recoveries at the population level is given by the product of γ and the number of infectious individuals, and so equals γI. Since recovery is assumed to confer permanent immunity, there is no flow out of the recovered class. This description of recovery leads to the following two additional equations:

$$\dot{I} = \beta SI/N - \gamma I \tag{2.2}$$

$$\dot{R} = \gamma I . \tag{2.3}$$

Equations 2.1 - 2.3, as a group, comprise the basic deterministic SIR model (see Figure 2.2).

This model does not include a description of vital dynamics — births and deaths are neglected. This may be a good approximation

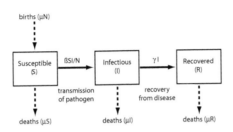

Figure 2.2 Basic structure of an SIR epidemic model. Dashed arrows show flows that are present only if vital dynamics are included.

if the duration of the epidemic is relatively short compared to the average lifespan of the population, as, for example, when modeling a single influenza epidemic in a human population. Since there are no births or deaths (and no influx or outflow of individuals), the total population size must be constant (as seen by summing up Equations 2.1 - 2.3). Thus, one of these equations is redundant and could be omitted. For instance, the number of recovereds is given by the total population size minus the numbers of susceptible and infectious individuals: $R = N - S - I$.

The SIR model (Equations 2.1 - 2.3) is often stated in terms of the fractions of the population that are found in each class. Many authors denote fractions by lowercase quantities. Since the lowercase i has a special mathematical meaning, the notation s, i, and r is typically avoided; instead, the susceptible, infectious, and recovered fractions are usually denoted x, y, and z. Since $x = S/N$, $y = I/N$, and $z = R/N$, the SIR model can be rewritten in terms of fractions as

$$\dot{x} = -\beta x y \tag{2.4}$$

$$\dot{y} = \beta x y - \gamma y \tag{2.5}$$

$$\dot{z} = \gamma y . \tag{2.6}$$

Notice that the denominator N is no longer present in this fraction-based representation.

2.2.1 Initial behavior of the SIR model

One of the primary questions of interest in epidemic modeling is whether an infection will spread upon introduction. Intuitively, this will happen if the initial infected individual is able to spread the infection to at least one susceptible individual, thereby maintaining or increasing the total number of infections. In the early stages of an epidemic, the population is almost entirely susceptible, so that $S \approx N$. The rate at which the first infectious individual gives rise to new infections is approximately equal to β, and so the nonlinear term $\beta SI/N$ can be approximated by the linear term βI. Since the average duration of infectiousness is $1/\gamma$ time units, the average number of secondary infections caused by the introduction of the single infectious individual into the otherwise entirely susceptible population is the product of the infection rate and the duration of infection, or

$$R_0 = \frac{\beta}{\gamma}. \qquad (2.7)$$

This important quantity has been given a special name, the basic reproductive number (Heesterbeek and Dietz, 1996; Macdonald, 1952). If R_0 is greater than one, then the initial case gives rise, on average, to more than one additional case, guaranteeing that the introduction of infection into an otherwise fully susceptible population will lead to the occurrence of an epidemic. If R_0 is less than one, then the initial cases are unable to replace themselves fully and the infection will die out.[2] Because it represents the boundary between a no-epidemic situation and an epidemic, the value $R_0 = 1$ is often referred to as the epidemic threshold.

The basic reproductive number is of such importance in predicting the possibility of epidemic spread following introduction of an infection into a susceptible population that it is common practice to attempt to determine the functional form of this quantity early in the analysis of a new epidemic model. Although this is often straightforward in simple situations, in more complex model settings it may be much more difficult to find analytical forms that specify the relevant parameter combinations (see, for instance, Diekmann et al., 1990). However, it can usually be shown numerically that there is some quantity that governs epidemic threshold behavior. In other

---

[2]The formulation of R_0 given in Equation 2.7 is specific to the SIR model given by Equations 2.1 - 2.3. As is evident throughout this book, however, the term basic reproductive number and the notation R_0 are used for analogous formulations found in other epidemic models.

words, for many models it can be shown that there is some combination of parameters whose value determines whether an epidemic can develop or not.

Further analysis of Equations 2.1 - 2.3, using the linear approximation βI for the transmission term, shows that during the initial stage of the epidemic, the number of infectious individuals grows exponentially at a rate r, where

$$r = \gamma(R_0 - 1). \tag{2.8}$$

Of course, exponential growth cannot continue for too long, as new infections will quickly deplete the number of susceptibles.

The basic reproductive number, R_0, only describes the average number of secondary infections at the beginning of an epidemic, when $S \approx N$. During the course of an epidemic, the number of susceptible individuals changes and is generally not near N, necessitating a different formulation to describe the average number of secondary infections due to a single infectious individual. The general reproductive number, R_t, fills this role — it describes the average number of secondary infections due to a single infectious individual at any time over the course of an epidemic. When there are S susceptibles remaining in the population, each infectious individual gives rise to new infections at a rate $\beta S/N$. Thus, R_t is given by the product of R_0 and S/N, the fraction of the population remaining susceptible at that time. As the number of susceptibles in the model given by Equations 2.1 - 2.3 becomes sufficiently depleted, R_t will fall below one and the number of infectious individuals will start to decline. Note that this will always happen in this model because the population size is constant and recovery is permanent so that a recovered individual can never leave that state.

As we will show below, these dynamics are not characteristic of all epidemic models. For example, simply adding vital dynamics (births and deaths) to the basic SIR model can allow a disease to be maintained in a population at an endemic level because the supply of susceptible individuals is continually renewed through births.

In this particular case it is straightforward to obtain an expression for the fraction of individuals who ever experience infection over the course of the epidemic, written f_∞. In the classic paper describing the basic SIR model, Kermack and McKendrick (1927) showed that the total size of the epidemic satisfies the relationship

$$f_\infty = 1 - \exp\left(-R_0 f_\infty\right). \tag{2.9}$$

Notice that $f_\infty = 0$ is always a solution of Equation 2.9. When R_0 is less than one, $f_\infty = 0$ is the only biologically relevant solution (there is an additional negative solution). When R_0 is greater than one, there is a positive solution, as expected since $R_0 > 1$ allows the occurrence of an epidemic.

2.2.2   Alternative descriptions of the transmission term

The basic reproductive number for the SIR model formulated above is independent of the size of the population, with R_0 equaling β/γ. This behavior arises because it was assumed that individuals made a fixed number of contacts, c, per unit time; in particular, the contact rate was assumed not to vary with population size, N. In turn, this assumption led to the transmission term being equal to $\beta SI/N$. This form of the transmission term is often known as standard incidence.

The number of contacts made by an individual need not be independent of N. Different assumptions about the dependence of c on N give rise to different forms of the transmission term and lead to R_0 having a dependence on the population size. The mass action incidence assumption takes the contact rate to be proportional to N. This corresponds to replacing c by cN in the above discussion, giving rise to the mass action transmission term βSI and the basic reproductive number equaling $\beta N/\gamma$.

The appropriate form for the transmission term depends both on the infection and on the setting of interest. In small populations, it is plausible that the contact rate would increase with the size of the population, but it is almost certainly the case that the number of effective contacts reaches a maximum level due to time constraints and the local nature of most behavioral interactions. Consequently, Dietz (1982) suggested that a more reasonable form for the contact rate would be the saturating function $cN/(N_s + N)$, where N_s is the value of N at which the contact rate takes half its ultimate value. This saturation function behaves like the mass action term when N is small, but like the standard incidence term when N becomes large, with the parameter N_s setting the scale on which saturation occurs.

Many studies of disease transmission in populations of moderate to large sizes have shown that R_0 either has no noticeable trend (Bjørnstad et al., 2002) as population size varies, or has a very slow increase with N (Anderson, 1982). For this reason, the standard incidence term is widely employed.

The issue of different forms for transmission and their relative merits is one that has appeared on several occasions in the infectious disease literature (Antonovics et al., 1995; Begon et al., 2002; de Jong et al., 1995; McCallum et al., 2001). Unfortunately, different authors have employed different terminologies and so the potential for confusion is rife. The issue is further complicated by the formulation of many models (particularly for the spread of infectious diseases in wildlife populations) in terms of the densities of individuals. Particularly in the ecological literature, the standard incidence form of transmission is also known as frequency dependent transmission, whereas the mass action form of transmission is also known as density dependent transmission.

De Jong et al. (1995) argue that the transmission term should be formulated in terms of densities. A confusing and unfortunate upshot of their argument is that they dub what is now generally termed standard incidence "true mass action" and what is now generally termed mass action incidence "pseudo mass action." Several more recent papers have questioned their reasoning (e.g., Begon et al., 2002; McCallum et al., 2001) and warn strongly against the use of de Jong et al.'s terminology. Both papers demonstrate the need to use caution in the formulation of transmission terms, and in distinguishing between numbers and densities.

2.3 DEMOGRAPHY AND EPIDEMIC MODELS

Unless a disease outbreak is short-lived in comparison to the timescale on which members of the population are born or die (the demographic timescale), demographic processes can have a significant impact on the fate on an infection. Most strikingly, the replenishment of susceptible individuals by birth can, as we shall see below, lead to the maintenance of an infection within a population. Most epidemiological models must, therefore, contain a description of at least some aspects of the demography of the population under consideration.

Most commonly, the demographic processes considered include only births and deaths, but, depending on the purpose of the model, migration, age structure, or other factors may also be incorporated. For example, because mortality from HIV/AIDS in developing countries is particularly high for individuals of reproductive age, studies of the impact of HIV/AIDS on the population age and sex distributions in countries of the developing world must include age-dependent descriptions of both disease transmission and demography (Anderson et al., 1988, 1989; Anderson and May, 1991).

Most epidemic models can be easily modified to include vital dynamics (births and deaths). The simplest way to do this is to assume that the birth rate is proportional to the total population size. The per capita birth rate is often written as μ, and so the number of births in the population equals μN. Furthermore, in many cases it is also assumed that the total population size remains constant and so the death rate is set equal to the birth rate. In these models, the average lifespan, L, is given by $1/\mu$.

2.3.1 The SIR model with vital dynamics

In the basic SIR model with vital dynamics all individuals are assumed to be susceptible at birth. For nonfatal diseases, it is assumed that the death rate does not depend on disease status, so that individuals in all classes experience the same per-capita death rate (see Figure 2.2). These assumptions lead to the following set of equations:

$$\dot{S} = \mu N - \beta SI/N - \mu S \qquad (2.10)$$

$$\dot{I} = \beta SI/N - (\gamma + \mu)I \qquad (2.11)$$

$$\dot{R} = \gamma I - \mu R. \qquad (2.12)$$

The behavior of this model is also governed by the basic reproductive number, which is now given by the expression $R_0 = \beta/(\mu + \gamma)$. Notice the slight difference between this expression and the corresponding expression for the SIR model without vital dynamics (Equation 2.7). Since individuals can die, the death rate slightly reduces the average duration of infectiousness. (If the average duration of infectiousness is short compared to the average lifespan, then $\gamma \gg \mu$, and this correction term is small.)

As in the SIR model without vital dynamics, an epidemic will occur if $R_0 > 1$. But remember that in the original model, eventually the supply of susceptibles becomes insufficient to maintain the infection, causing it to die out. Unlike the closed population, however, when the population is open due to the incorporation of births and deaths, the replenishment of the susceptible population by births allows for maintenance of infection. When $R_0 > 1$, there is a stable endemic equilibrium at which there is a balance both between the birth of susceptibles and their loss (by death and infection), and between the generation of new infections and their loss (by recovery and death) of infectious individuals (Hethcote, 1974). This equilibrium is globally attracting, meaning that the population distribution will always approach this equlibrium. Notice that because the number of infectious individuals is at steady state, the general reproductive number, R_t, is equal to one at equilibrium. The numbers of susceptible and infectious individuals at this equilibrium, written S^* and I^*, are given by

$$S^* = \frac{N}{R_0} \quad \text{and} \quad I^* = \frac{\mu N (R_0 - 1)}{\beta}. \qquad (2.13)$$

An important observation is that the fraction of the population that remains susceptible at the equilibrium equals the reciprocal of R_0. Furthermore, for this simple deterministic model, the threshold condition $R_0 > 1$ again ensures both disease invasion and disease persistence.

2.4   MORE COMPLEX MODELS

Analysis of the SIR model given by Equations 2.1 - 2.3 or by Equations 2.10 - 2.11 has resulted in important general insights about how, when, and why epidemics spread in a population. Nonetheless, the models are built upon a number of assumptions that often provide a poor description of real-world epidemiological situations, limiting their practical value. Consequently, a wide variety of more complex models that alter one or more of these assumptions have been developed.

   In the following we discuss some of the most common choices made in model formulation and the ways in which additional complexity is incorporated. The choices and complexities we discuss include 1) whether the population is described in terms of its individual members or in terms of the numbers of individuals in each infection class, 2) more complex descriptions of how the disease progresses through time, 3) allowing for randomness in the epidemiological processes, 4) whether time is measured continuously or in discrete units, 5) more sophisticated descriptions of the mixing of individuals within and among populations, and 6) time-varying transmission rates. In light of our discussion of these complexities, at the end of this chapter we revisit the concept of the basic reproductive number, R_0.

2.4.1   Individual-based and population-level models

In mathematical descriptions of disease processes, individuals are described by their state — those features that determine their potential to acquire and transmit infection. At the very least, the state of individuals reflects their infection status, such as whether they are susceptible to the infection, infectious, or recovered from infection. Depending on the level of detail of the model, other features, such as age, spatial location, genetic, and behavioral factors, might also be required to specify the states of individuals. Many epidemiological models employ highly simplified descriptions of the disease process, and so in many cases models only distinguish between a small number of possible states.

Because the spread of an infection within the model depends on the states of each of its members, the model must account for these states. This can be achieved in one of two fundamentally different ways: at the level of the population or at the level of the individual (Cushing, 1998; DeAngelis and Gross, 1992; Diekmann et al., 1998b; Metz and Diekmann, 1986). Population-level models, such as the SIR model described above, keep track of the total numbers of individuals in each state, but do not explicitly model individuals and their specific behaviors. They assume that populations are large enough that the effects of deviations from the mean can be ignored when considering the infection process at the population level. In effect, this allows one to treat the population as if every individual is identical and equivalent to the average individual, even though there is underlying variability in the population. In such a model, transitions from one state to another are determined by rates of flow between states and the total number of individuals in the source state. Details concerning the specific individuals within states are not taken into account explicitly. In addition, population-based compartment models, such as the basic SIR model, allow for fractional "individuals" to flow from one compartment to another, a situation that is obviously unrealistic.

Individual-based approaches, on the other hand, explicitly model each individual, keeping track of the state of each member of the population and of underlying characteristics associated with those individuals (such as level of susceptibility or specific risk behaviors), and so, in general, they can more easily address the impact of heterogeneity among individuals. In addition, because individuals are explicitly considered, such models do not have the unrealistic attribute of fractional individuals. To illustrate the general approach of individual-based models, we describe here an individual-based SIR model that is analogous to the basic population-level SIR model; in later chapters we will discuss individual-based applications to the study of specific infectious diseases.

2.4.1.1 An individual-based SIR model

Figure 2.3 compares the basic structure of an individual-based SIR model and a population-based SIR model. In the individual-based SIR model, all N individuals within the population are considered explicitly. Individuals are classified according to their infection status — susceptible, infectious, or recovered — and changes in infection status are monitored on a daily basis. Individuals are assumed to make a daily average of c contacts with randomly chosen members of the population. These encounters are simulated by drawing pairs of individuals at random from the population. Infection can occur if an encounter occurs between a susceptible individual and an infectious individual. In the simplest models, the probability that infection occurs during such an encounter is assumed to be a constant, p, although this assumption is easily relaxed. In addition, the simplest models assume that once infection occurs, an individual remains infectious exactly m days, at which time recovery occurs and the individual becomes permanently immune.

One difference between the individual-based model and the earlier population-based model is that the individual-based model treats time as a discretely varying quantity, tracking changes on a daily basis (or other desired time unit), as opposed to the flows of the compartmental model that occur continuously in time. The model is described in terms of the properties and behavior of each individual at each time unit, rather than specifying the behavior in terms of the total numbers of susceptible and infectious individuals as is the case with the population-based model. In addition, the individual-based model allows for the situation where transmission, by chance, may not occur even though contact occurs between a susceptible individual and an infectious individual. This random effect can be incorporated into population-based models, but it is not a feature of the basic SIR compartmental model described above.

The population-level approach has tended to dominate the epidemiological literature because it generates simple models with limited numbers of parameters (e.g., a low-dimensional set of ordinary differential equations) that are amenable both to mathematical analysis and numerical simulation. The basic SIR model given in Equations 2.1 - 2.3 and other models that use a similar compartmental structure are probably the most common population-level models in mathematical epidemiology.

The individual-based approach typically leads to more complex models with larger numbers of parameters and which are often better

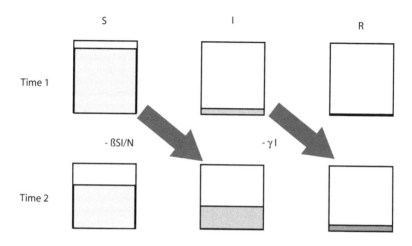

S I R

Time 1

Time 2

- ßSI/N -γI

A population-based SIR model

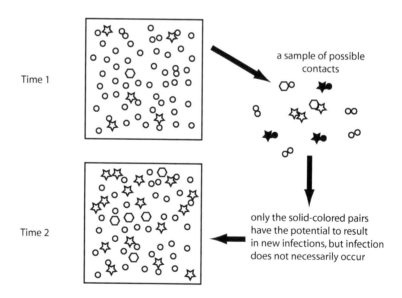

Time 1

Time 2

a sample of possible contacts

only the solid-colored pairs have the potential to result in new infections, but infection does not necessarily occur

An individual-based SIR model

Figure 2.3 A comparison of a population-based and an individual-based SIR model. Arrows in the top diagram represent flows between compartments with the indicated flow rates. In the bottom diagram circles represent susceptible individuals, stars represent infectious individuals, and hexagons represent recovered individuals.

suited for simulation than analysis. Since the description is at the level of the individual, simulation is often computationally expensive, particularly when population sizes are large. Given their inherent complexity, individual-based model formulations often include much more detailed and realistic descriptions of disease processes than do population-level models. In addition, because of their focus on the individual, such models almost always incorporate random (stochastic) effects, while, as discussed below, population-level models can be of either type.

With the increasing availability of high-powered computers, individual-based approaches are gaining in popularity. Several computer programs exist that provide environments in which individual-based models can easily be developed and simulated numerically. While some of these programs are designed specifically for epidemiological settings (for example, the GERMS package developed by Koopman et al. (2000)), others provide a more general individual-based modeling framework, including AnyLogic (XJ Technologies Company, see website at http://www.xjtek.com) and Repast (for a description of this program see North et al. (2006) or the project homepage at http://repast.sourceforge.net).

It is important to understand that in both population-level and individual-level contexts, the "individual" need not represent a single member of the population. As an example, transmission might be modeled at the level of a family: when a disease is highly transmissible, the introduction of infection into a household by one family member might lead to all family members becoming infected. In such cases, a population-level model might track the number of susceptible and infectious families, while individual-level models might account for the disease state of each family in the population.

2.4.2 Descriptions of the disease process

Most epidemiological models employ a highly simplified description of the disease process within an individual, both in terms of possible disease states (susceptible, infectious, recovered, etc.) and characteristics related to those states, such as length of time spent within one state or state-related factors influencing disease transmission. These disease states are described from the viewpoint of transmission — the infectious class refers to those individuals who can transmit infection — but as discussed at the beginning of this chapter, this might not correspond exactly to those who are exhibiting symptoms. This distinction can be important when comparing real-world incidence data, which is likely to reflect those individuals who exhibit symptoms, with model behavior. For example, the patterns of infectiousness and symptoms may be quite different for diseases with long incubation periods, such as HIV/AIDS. Additional disease states (e.g., infectious but not exhibiting symptoms, or infectious and exhibiting symptoms) can be included to accommodate such distinctions, at the expense of an increase in the complexity of the model.

One common assumption related to the disease process is that there is a fixed rate of recovery. This corresponds to assuming that the duration of infectiousness is exponentially distributed, with mean $1/\gamma$ (Cox and Miller, 1965). This assumption is a poor description of the recovery process: in reality, the chance of recovery (per unit time) increases over the course of infection (Sartwell, 1950, 1966). This leads to individuals' infectious periods being more closely distributed about their mean than an exponential distribution because far fewer individuals recover long before or long after the mean infectious period than would be expected with a constant rate of recovery.

The fixed recovery rate assumption is usually made for mathematical convenience as it means that the model need not keep track of the times at which each infectious individual became infected. Recall that in the basic SIR model given by Equations 2.1 - 2.3 or by Equations 2.10 - 2.11, the term describing the recovery of infectious individuals was simply given by γI. Notice that this term depends only on the number of infectious individuals at the present time. (This reflects the so-called memoryless property of the exponential distribution (Cox and Miller, 1965).) Inclusion of more general descriptions of the recovery process requires a more complex form of the recovery term, involving some knowledge of the history of the system. In general, this leads to an infinite-dimensional model, which can be described in one of several ways, such as a partial differential equation (PDE) model, a delay-differential equation model, or an integral equation model (see, for example, Castillo-Chavez et al., 1989a,b; Grossman, 1980; Hethcote and Tudor, 1980; Hoppensteadt, 1974). The specific questions to be addressed by the model determine whether the increased complexity is justified.

Another common assumption of SIR models is that a newly infected individual becomes infectious immediately upon infection. Many diseases must, however, incubate within the body for some time before an infected individual becomes infectious. Adding an additional disease state, an exposed class, to the basic SIR model can allow for such a latent period between exposure to the infection and the start of infectiousness. The resulting model is commonly referred to as an

SEIR (susceptible/exposed/infectious/recovered) model (Wilson and Worcester, 1945a). As with the recovery period, the latent period is often described by an exponential distribution, but more general distributions can be modeled.

In reality, infectiousness is not generally a binary state where one is infectious or not. In most cases, individuals exhibit a degree of infectiousness that reflects the level of the infectious agent (such as a virus) within their bodies. In many cases, infectiousness will tend to increase as the virus replicates, before peaking and then decreasing (perhaps because the immune system overcomes the virus, or because the virus kills the individual). As before, since an individual's infectiousness depends on the time since acquiring infection, the model must include some knowledge of the history of the system and so general descriptions of time-varying infectiousness again lead to an infinite-dimensional model (Blythe and Anderson, 1988; Cairns, 1990). Interestingly, the model of Kermack and McKendrick (1927), the earliest and perhaps the most important of the basic SIR models, included variable infectiousness within its formulation, and so Kermack and McKendrick's expression for the total size of an epidemic in a closed population (Equation 2.9) actually applies to a more general situation than our earlier discussion indicated (see the discussion of Diekmann et al., 1995).

One simple way to include a more general description of the time course of infection within the compartmental model framework is to introduce additional disease stages (Bailey, 1964; Cox and Miller, 1965; Jensen, 1948; Longini et al., 1989). These stages can sometimes be chosen to correspond to actual disease states, although in most cases these stages are merely a mathematical device. This approach can be used to describe infectious periods that are not exponentially distributed; in fact, a family of distributions known as the gamma distribution can be easily parameterized in this fashion (Anderson and Watson, 1980; Andersson and Britton, 2000b; Bailey, 1964; Jensen, 1948; Lloyd, 2001a; Malice and Kryscio, 1989; Nisbet and Gurney, 1986). This technique can also be used to approximate variable infectiousness by assuming that individuals in the different infectious stages have different levels of infectiousness (Longini et al., 1989).

The inadequacy of the standard description of constant infectiousness over an exponentially distributed infectious period has long been appreciated for diseases, such as HIV/AIDS, that have long and often variable incubation periods. The pathology of HIV is particularly interesting as the virus load shows a large, but short-lived, peak during primary infection, then remains at a fairly low, steady level for the long asymptomatic phase, before increasing during the symptomatic AIDS phase (Pantaleo et al., 1993). The multiple-stage approach has been used successfully in many models of HIV/AIDS transmission (for example, Hethcote, 1989; Hyman and Stanley, 1988; Jacquez et al., 1988; Longini et al., 1989).

Given the additional complexity of individual-based models, it is somewhat ironic that it is often easier to include general descriptions of infectious periods within the individual-based framework. For many individual-based simulation codes, the time at which an individual will recover is determined at the time of infection by drawing a number from the distribution of infectious periods. For such simulation codes, it is a straightforward matter to draw this number from a general, rather than exponential, distribution. Unfortunately, the additional complexity introduced by the consideration of variable infectiousness is also an issue for the individual-based approach because, at each time point, the chance of transmission between an infectious-susceptible pair depends on the time since infection, necessitating that the model keep track of this additional parameter.

2.4.3 The impact of random factors — deterministic vs. stochastic models

One of the assumptions of the simple SIR model given by Equations 2.1 - 2.3 or by Equations 2.10 - 2.11 is that random effects have no impact on the system. Models that make such an assumption are called deterministic models, as their behavior is entirely determined by the configuration of the system at a given time. Because of this, if a numerical simulation of the deterministic model is rerun beginning from the same initial conditions, exactly the same outcome will be observed. An important additional feature of deterministic approaches is that they model the number of individuals in a given state as a continuously varying quantity. When the number of disease states is finite, a deterministic model can be represented as a set of ordinary differential equations describing the rates at which movement between different states occurs (as in Equations 2.1 - 2.3).

Deterministic models are often amenable to mathematical analysis, and even though complete solutions are only available for the simplest of these models, qualitative and quantitative features of their behavior can often be described. Simulation of deterministic models is usually straightforward, particularly for models consisting of ordinary differential equations (see, for instance, Press et al., 1996). For these reasons, they have been used widely in epidemic modeling studies, and they have provided important insights into the nature of epidemic spread within and among populations. Nevertheless, the real world is not deterministic — random factors abound and are often important during the disease process.

Models that account for random effects are known as stochastic models. The individual-based model described in Section 2.4.1 is stochastic since it accounts for random encounters between specific pairs of individuals and for randomness in the process of transmission between infectious and susceptible individuals.

Randomness makes each simulation run (or realization) of a stochastic model different, even if the same set of initial conditions is used; this is quite distinct from the behavior of a deterministic model. Repeated simulation of a stochastic model using the same starting conditions leads to the generation of a set of different realizations of the model. Analysis of these results involves statistical analysis of the characteristics of the distribution of particular model outcomes with the entire set of model realizations. Properties of these distributions can then be discussed. For example, in some simulation runs a disease will succeed in invading a population, in some runs it will not only invade, but it will persist, and in yet other runs it may not take off at all. Analysis of the entire set of model realizations allows determination of a variety of outcomes, such as the probability that a disease can invade or persist in a given situation or the average number of cases predicted to occur following disease introduction (see, for example, Whittle, 1955).

A fundamental random effect is demographic stochasticity, which arises because the population consists of a finite number of individuals (Bartlett, 1960b; Nisbet and Gurney, 1982; Renshaw, 1991). Particularly in small populations, disease transmission can be subject to relatively large random effects. A common consequence of this kind of process is an interruption in the chain of infection (as would happen if the last remaining infected individual recovers before passing on the disease) and hence extinction of a disease within a population (Bartlett, 1956, 1957, 1960a, 1964; Black, 1966). A well-known weakness of many deterministic models is their inability to capture such extinction events — in such models numbers of infectives can often recover despite falling to levels at which tiny fractions of individuals are infected (Bolker and Grenfell, 1993; Grenfell, 1992). A stochastic framework is necessary in order to realistically model such behavior. A stochastic framework must also be employed if a population is to be treated as a collection of discrete individuals, even if the population is infinite in size, since deterministic models assume continuous flows between classes and so necessarily involve fractional numbers of individuals.

Other stochastic effects can also have an impact upon an epidemiological system. For example, climatic conditions might affect the transmission of an infectious agent, perhaps because weather patterns alter behavioral patterns of the population (for instance, cold weather might lead people to congregate indoors) or because the infectious agent might be less likely to survive outside of its host under certain conditions. An important property of such environmental stochasticity (and one that differs from the randomness introduced by demographic stochasticity) is that it is likely to be autocorrelated — the weather conditions at a certain time influence and can be used to predict, at least in the short term, those in the future. Because of this, the randomness caused by environmental fluctuations is poorly modeled by white noise alone (a standard way to deal mathematically with random effects), as such a noise term exhibits no autocorrelation. Turelli (1977) provides a discussion of the population-level impact of autocorrelated noise, highlighting the important differences that arise between models that represent environmental fluctuations as white noise and those that employ autocorrelated noise.

Stochastic effects are clearly most important when population sizes (or the sizes of certain subpopulations) are small. One setting in which random effects can have a major impact is during the early stages of an outbreak: invasion of an infection is a highly random process, particularly if there are only a small number of initial infectious individuals (see Section 2.4.3.3 for a discussion how one analysis technique for stochastic models, branching processes, is used to address the question of pathogen invasion).

More generally, it is important to realize that the context will influence whether a population of a particular size is small enough for stochastic effects to play a major role. Before the introduction of mass vaccination programs in the years following World War II, childhood diseases, such as measles, exhibited large-scale recurrent epidemics in the major cities of Europe and America. As the number of infectious individuals fell to low levels in the waning days of an epidemic, local extinction, known as disease fadeout, often occurred due to the fact that transmission by the small number of infectious individuals just didn't happen because of chance events. This pattern was possible even when the number of susceptible individuals remained high and was frequently observed in all but the largest cities (Bartlett, 1956, 1957, 1960a, 1964; Keeling and Grenfell, 1997). This example illustrates how mathematical modeling studies have helped to elucidate potential underlying causes for the pattern of recurrent epidemics of childhood illnesses. In particular, they have helped to point out that large population sizes are no guarantee that stochastic factors can be ignored, and they have helped to test different hypotheses about the underlying factors leading to repeated epidemics within populations.

2.4.3.1 *The inclusion of stochastic effects in epidemic models*

The rate equations describing a deterministic model can be reinterpreted to give the probabilities of movement of individuals between different states (Bartlett, 1960b). For instance, in a stochastic analog of the deterministic SIR model (Equations 2.1 - 2.3), the infection term βSI would be interpreted as follows: the probability of an infection event occurring in the (short) time interval from t to $t + dt$ would be $\beta SI dt$. The simplest simulation approach would draw a random number to determine whether such an event occurred (assuming that a susceptible individual came into contact with an infectious individual), and if it had, the number of susceptibles would decrease by one and the number of infectious individuals would increase by one. A similar procedure could be employed to handle recovery events. These two steps form the basis of a Monte Carlo simulation method — so called because of its reliance on the drawing of random numbers.

Several exact Monte Carlo techniques are used to simulate epidemic models (Bartlett, 1956; Gibson and Bruck, 2000; Gillespie, 1977; Renshaw, 1991). These are based on the properties of the Poisson processes that underlie the stochastic formulation of the epidemic model (Cox and Miller, 1965). For a Poisson process occurring at a constant rate it can be shown that the time until the occurrence of the next event is exponentially distributed with mean given by the reciprocal of the rate. In the time up until the next event, the numbers of susceptible and infectious individuals will not change, so this argument can be applied to the infection and recovery processes separately. Numbers can be drawn from the two exponential distributions describing the time until the next infection or recovery event. By finding the smallest of these times, the next event (recovery or infection) can be determined and the populations updated appropriately.

An alternative technique makes use of the fact that the sum of two independent Poisson processes is also a Poisson process, with rate given by the sum of those of the two separate Poisson processes. For the SIR model, the time until the next event of either kind can therefore be found by sampling from an exponential distribution with the mean equal to the reciprocal of the sum of the recovery and infection rates. It then remains to determine which of the two events occurred. The relative probabilities of the next event being infection or recovery is given by the relative sizes of the two rates: for example, if the infection rate is twice the recovery rate, the probability that the next event will be an infection is 2/3 while the recovery probability is 1/3. Which of the events occurs can be determined by drawing a random number that is uniformly distributed between 0 and 1.

A general stochastic model would have more than two possible events occurring at any timestep. The first approach just described requires as many random numbers to be drawn at each step as there are events, whereas the second approach only requires two, one to determine when the next event occurs and a second to determine what type of event occurred.

Since exact Monte Carlo methods simulate each transition or event separately, they can be computationally expensive in terms of time, particularly when the population size is large. As will be illustrated in later chapters, this fact is an important constraint that may sometimes limit the usefulness of many individual-based models in addressing real problems.

Notice that these Monte Carlo techniques model discrete individuals. In the stochastic differential equation (SDE) approach, the number of individuals in a given state is modeled as a continuously varying quantity, as in the deterministic model, but a random noise term is added to the rate equations (Karatzas and Shreve, 1991; Øksendal, 1998). (See Kloeden and Platen (1999) for a discussion of numerical techniques for the simulation of SDEs, which are also discussed, at an introductory level, in Higham (2001)). This approach can mimic the effects of stochasticity, often successfully for moderately sized populations, but it suffers from the same "lack of extinction despite small numbers" effect previously described for the deterministic model. Mathematical analysis may, however, be possible within the SDE approach.

2.4.3.2 Strategies used in the analysis of stochastic epidemic models

The mathematical analysis of stochastic models tends to be much more involved than that of their deterministic counterparts, and a number of analytic techniques have been developed to aid in their study. These include branching process theory (Jagers, 1975; Taneyhill et al., 1999), stochastic differential equation theory (Doering, 1991; Karatzas and Shreve, 1991; Øksendal, 1998), and martingale theory (Andersson and Britton, 2000a; Becker, 1993). Jagers (1975) and Doering (1991) are accessible introductions to branching processes and stochastic differential equations, respectively.

While these techniques are difficult to use in general, they have provided many useful insights. For example, there is a large body of theory on the impact of stochastic effects on the invasion of infection. This theory has developed in large part because early in a disease outbreak (when the invasion is occurring) almost the entire population is susceptible and, as discussed earlier, in such a situation the system can be treated as if it were linear. The linearity of the system makes analysis of the models much simpler. The most important results about disease invasion in stochastic models are analogs of the $R_0 = 1$ invasion threshold of the deterministic SIR model. Analyses show that even if R_0 is greater than one, invasion of an infection is not guaranteed in a stochastic setting: with a small initial pool of infectious individuals, there is some chance that they will all recover before passing on the infection. Furthermore, as the initial pool of infectious individuals increases in size, stochastic extinction becomes less likely.

2.4.3.3 Branching process theory and invasion dynamics

An important consequence of the assumption that the disease system can be represented as a linear process early in an epidemic is that the numbers of secondary infections of different individuals are statistically independent. (This would not be the case in the full nonlinear model, since secondary infections of one individual would reduce the pool of available susceptibles, potentially reducing the number of secondary infections of other individuals.) Branching process theory in combination with this assumption of linearity can be used to derive the probability that a disease will become extinct or will persist within a population.

The theory centers around the distribution of the number of secondary infections that are due to a given infectious individual. Let q_k denote the probability that an infectious individual gives rise to k secondary infections. If each individual gave rise to exactly x secondary infections, we would have that $q_x = 1$ and all the other q_k would equal zero. Different model assumptions give rise to different distributions of secondary infections. For the stochastic analog of the SIR model discussed above, in which recovery occurs at a constant rate γ and secondary infections are being produced at rate β over the infectious period, it can be shown that the number of secondary infections follows a geometric distribution, with

$$q_k = \frac{\gamma \beta^k}{(\gamma + \beta)^{k+1}}.$$

(2.14)

This distribution has mean equal to β/γ: the average number of secondary infections is given by the R_0 of the deterministic model. If, on the other hand, recovery is taken to occur exactly $1/\gamma$ time units after infection, the number of secondary infections can be shown to follow a Poisson distribution, with mean β/γ.

The distribution of secondary infections can be summarized by the probability generating function

$$G(t) = \sum_{k=0}^{\infty} q_k t^k.$$

(2.15)

This is a power series in the variable t, where the coefficients of the various powers of t are equal to the q_k. Generating functions have several well-known properties, many of which explain their utility in statistical and probability theory. For instance, the value of dG/dt, evaluated at $t = 1$, gives the average number of secondary infections. Values of the higher-order derivatives of $G(t)$, evaluated at $t = 1$, can be used to calculate higher-order moments (such as the variance) of the distribution. Notice that the value of $G(1)$ is equal to one since it is the sum of the q_k.

The central result of branching process theory is that the infection process either goes extinct or continues forever. (Keep in mind that the branching process theory applies to the linearized epidemic model for which the supply of susceptibles is unlimited.) The probability of eventual extinction, if there is a single initial infectious individual, is given by the smallest nonnegative solution of

$$G(t) = t.$$

(2.16)

Since we know that $G(1) = 1$, this solution satisfies $0 \leq t \leq 1$.

For the stochastic analog of the SIR model outlined above, with the q_k given in Equation 2.14, it can be shown that the generating function is given by $G(t) = \gamma/(\gamma - \beta(t-1))$. The smallest nonnegative root of Equation 2.16 depends on the value of $R_0 = \beta/\gamma$. If the basic reproductive number is less than one, the root is equal to one, whereas if $R_0 > 1$ the root is equal to $1/R_0$. The branching process either goes extinct or grows indefinitely, and the extinction probability equals 1 or $1/R_0$, depending on whether $R_0 < 1$ or $R_0 > 1$, respectively. When there is more than one initial infectious individual, extinction of the branching process occurs with probability 1 or $(1/R_0)^{I_0}$, where I_0 denotes the initial number of infectious individuals. This result follows as a consequence of the independence property discussed above.

Of course, the number of infectious individuals cannot continue to grow in the full nonlinear model. Over time, the number of susceptibles is depleted and the linear approximation becomes a poor description of reality. But by this time, the number of infectious individuals is likely large enough that stochastic extinction is unlikely to occur until after a significant outbreak has occurred. The outcomes of the branching process analysis are reinterpreted in the nonlinear model as follows: either a major outbreak occurs (corresponding to unbounded growth in the branching process model) or a minor outbreak occurs (corresponding to extinction in the branching process model). Thus, the solution to Equation 2.16 gives the probability of occurrence of a minor outbreak in the nonlinear model.

For the stochastic analog of the SIR model outlined above, it can be shown that the generating function is given by $G(t) = \gamma/(\gamma - \beta(t-1))$. This leads to the famous result that the probability of a minor outbreak is equal to one if R_0 is below one. When R_0 is above one, a minor outbreak occurs with probability $(1/R_0)^{I_0}$, while a major outbreak occurs with probability $1 - (1/R_0)^{I_0}$. Again, I_0 is the initial number of infectious individuals.

2.4.3.4 *More generally...*

A number of other techniques have been used to give insight into the behavior of stochastic models. For example, it is sometimes possible to use coupling methods, in which the behavior of an analytically intractable model is bounded by that of two mathematically tractable models (Andersson and Britton, 2000a; Ball, 1995). In other words, the behavior of the original model must fall between the behaviors exhibited by the two models that can be analyzed.

Because of the difficulty in analyzing stochastic models, mathematical analysis is often replaced or supplemented by Monte Carlo simulation techniques that are used to generate simulation runs, or realizations, of the model (Bartlett, 1956; Gibson and Bruck, 2000; Gillespie, 1977; Renshaw, 1991). As discussed before, stochastic effects lead to variation between realizations of the model, even in the case when all realizations are started at the same set of initial conditions.

An alternative way of describing the behavior of a stochastic model is in terms of the moments (e.g., mean, variance, skewness) of the distribution of realizations. The deterministic model attempts to model the mean of this distribution, but it gives no information about higher-order moments. Higher-order moments are of obvious interest when making predictions of the future time course of an epidemic, as the variance describes the variability of realizations about their mean, and can be used to suggest confidence intervals for such predictions. Variability about the mean can also be used as a measure of the likelihood of persistence of a disease (see, for example, Keeling, 2000a,b; Nisbet and Gurney, 1982) — extinction is unlikely to occur if individual realizations remain close to their mean.

It is possible to develop sets of differential equations, known as moment equations, that model the time evolution of the second- and higher-order moments (Isham, 1991; Keeling, 2000a,b; Lloyd, 2004; Whittle, 1957). The moment equations can be used to estimate variability without recourse to numerical simulation of the full stochastic model, which can often be a computationally expensive task, particularly when the population size is large. The development of moment equations, however, is complicated by nonlinearities in the system. Nonlinear terms lead to coupling between moment equations of different orders. For example, the equations for the means might involve variances and covariances in addition to the means themselves. In such cases, the moment equations do not form a closed set, and, apart from the rare cases in which the infinite set can be solved, a moment closure technique must be employed to produce a useful (finite) description of the system.

Several moment closure approximations have been suggested, most of which assume that the distribution of realizations follows some known distribution, such as the multivariate normal (MVN) distribution (Whittle, 1957). A relationship that exists between the moments of the given distribution can then be imposed upon the moment equations. For instance, because the third-order central moments of an MVN are zero, the multivariate normal moment approximation imposes this constraint on the moment equations, leading to a closed set of equations for orders one and two. Techniques such as this are becoming increasingly important analytical tools within mathematical epidemiology (see, for example, Bauch, 2002; Bolker and Pacala, 1997; Keeling, 2000a).

2.4.3.5 *Stochasticity in the SIR model with demography*

As discussed in Section 2.3, when births and deaths are included in the deterministic SIR model, the condition $R_0 > 1$ ensures both successful invasion of the infection upon its introduction and persistence of the infection. The behavior is slightly more complex for stochastic formulations of this model. As previously discussed, random effects lead to variability in the behavior of realizations of the process, even when started from the same initial conditions (Isham, 1991; Lloyd, 2004). As we have already seen, random effects mean that disease invasion is no longer certain even when R_0 is greater than one. Stochastic effects also impact upon the persistence of the infection.

Stochastic effects prevent the system from settling into equilibrium — individual realizations continue to fluctuate around the level predicted by the deterministic model (Aparicio and Solari, 2001b; Bartlett, 1956; Lloyd, 2004; Nåsell, 1999). Approximation techniques (such as the moment equations mentioned above) can be used to predict the size of these fluctuations, and it is found that the coefficient of variation of the number of infectious individuals, defined as the standard deviation of the fluctuations in the number of infectious individuals divided by the mean number of infectious individuals, scales as the reciprocal of the square root of the population size (Bartlett, 1956, 1960b; Lloyd, 2004; Nåsell, 1999; Schenzle and Dietz, 1987). (This result has some correspondence with the central limit theorem of statistics; see Kurtz (1970, 1971).) Notice that if these fluctuations are sufficiently large, then the number of infectious individuals can come close to zero and hence the disease can undergo extinction, even though $R_0 > 1$. This endemic fadeout effect (Bartlett, 1956, 1957, 1960a, 1964; Black, 1966) has received much attention in the setting of childhood diseases such as measles.

2.4.4 Continuous time vs. discrete time formulations

Real epidemic processes clearly operate in continuous time, but in many cases it is reasonable for models of those processes to operate over discrete time units, such as days or weeks. Our example individual-based model, for instance, employed a day-by-day description of the epidemic process. The most common reason for employing a discrete time model is that the relevant epidemiological data are available in discrete time form, such as reports of the weekly numbers of cases. Discrete time processes are also, in some cases, simpler to analyze and simulate.

The choice of an appropriate discrete time step is of critical importance in these models. The time step must be sufficiently short so that the rates of the different processes being modeled remain fairly constant over the time step — choosing overly long time steps can give misleading results. For example, imagine that a discrete time model assumes that the infection rate is constant over a given time interval but that the interval is long enough for many of the individuals to recover. The discrete time model has the clear potential to overestimate the infection rate.

An inappropriate temporal discretization can lead to oscillatory solutions that are just an artifact of the modeling technique or, in more extreme cases, population numbers in the model can become negative (see, for example, the discussion on pp. 27-28 and 195-197 in Diekmann and Heesterbeek, 2000). The epidemiological literature has provided several unfortunate examples in which apparently interesting behavior has later been traced to an inappropriate choice of time step. Anderson and May (1991), for instance, suggest that some of the findings of Knox (1980) are dependent on the choice of a one year time step.

Even when a continuous time model is employed, simulation of that model often employs a discrete time approximation. For instance, numerical integration of a set of ordinary differential equations (such as Equations 2.1 - 2.3) using standard numerical techniques (Press et al., 1996) proceeds with the use of discrete time steps, although some techniques adapt the time step in an appropriate way to ensure accuracy. The stochastic Monte Carlo simulation technique discussed above employs a continuous time description as it models each individual event (e.g., the transition of an individual between two disease states) that occurs separately. An alternative stochastic simulation technique, which is often much faster, employs a fixed time step approach, assuming that the rates of each process remain constant over a short time interval (Aparicio and Solari, 2001a). Individual-based models can also be modeled using either discrete or continuous time approaches: in the former case, the states of each individual are updated simultaneously (synchronous updating), whereas in the latter, individuals' states are updated one at a time (asynchronous updating).

2.4.4.1 The chain binomial model

The most important discrete time epidemic model is the chain binomial model. Becker (1989) provides an excellent review of the structure, analysis, and use of this model. It employs a simple description of the time course of infection whereby individuals are assumed to undergo a latent period of fixed duration followed by a relatively short infectious period, which is modeled as an instantaneous event. Thus, a natural time step for the model is the generation time of infection, which, by assumption, is equal to the duration of the latent period.

The chain binomial model includes the assumption that contacts between susceptible and infectious individuals occur independently, and, in addition, the model assumes that each susceptible individual has the same chance of making an effective contact with any infectious individual who is present. The probability that a given susceptible escapes infection when exposed to the i infectious individuals of the current generation is written as q_i. Writing the numbers of susceptible and infectious individuals at time t as S_t and I_t, and ignoring births and deaths, we have that

$$Pr(I_{t+1} = x \,|\, S_t = s, I_t = i) = \frac{s!}{x!(s-x)!} \, (1-q_i)^x \, q_i^{s-x} \quad x = 0, 1, \ldots s.$$

(2.17)

Because infection either occurs or doesn't occur, at each time step, the number of infection events is described by a binomial distribution. Thus, the probability that describes whether the epidemic follows a particular time course, or epidemic chain, is given by multiplying terms from different binomial distributions. Notice that the change in the number of susceptibles in a given generation equals the number of infections that occurred.

Two different assumptions about the probabilities q_i have been made. The Reed-Frost model, first reported in the literature by Wilson and Burke (1942) (but see also Dietz and Schenzle (1985); Dietz (1988), and En'ko (1889)), assumes that $q_i = q^i$, which corresponds to assuming that the effective contacts of each infectious individual are independent. This somewhat resembles the situation envisaged in the mass action description of infection. The Greenwood model (Greenwood, 1931) assumes that $q_i = q$, when $i > 0$, and that $q_0 = 1$ — as long as there are any infectious individuals present, the chance of infection does not depend on the number of infectious individuals. This describes a situation in which disease transmission is saturated, and it is often used to describe a highly infectious disease in a family setting, when the chance of a single infectious individual passing on disease is sufficiently high that addition of extra infectious individuals would not increase the probability of transmission.

The formulation of chain binomial models facilitates statistical analysis, and allows parameter estimation and hypothesis testing to be carried out within a rigorous statistical framework (see Becker (1989)). For instance, because explicit expressions for the probability distribution of epidemic sizes in small group settings, such as households, can be obtained, statistical methods can be used to estimate parameters such as q using data from family studies (for an early example, see Heasman and Reid (1961)). Generalizations of these models, which include heterogeneity and time-varying transmission rates, can be used to test whether disease transmission exhibits significant heterogeneity (Becker and Hopper, 1983; Becker, 1989; Klauber and Angulo, 1976). One notable use of such models is provided by studies of the transmission dynamics of measles in Iceland, in which Cliff and co-workers employ a spatial variant of the chain binomial model (Cliff and Ord, 1978; Cliff et al., 1981).

2.4.5 Mixing patterns and other sources of variation in transmission rates

Disease transmission occurs when susceptible and infectious individuals meet in such a way that successful transmission occurs. The transmission process, therefore, depends on the mixing pattern of the population and details of the process by which a pathogen is passed from an infectious to a susceptible individual.

Both the standard incidence and mass action descriptions of transmission make two important assumptions. First, they assume that both the susceptible and infectious populations can be treated as if they are homogeneous groups, so that each susceptible is equally susceptible to the infection and each infectious individual is equally infectious. Second, they assume that the population is well mixed, meaning that any given individual has the same probability of contacting any other individual within the population.

Analysis of many data sets, however, has revealed evidence for heterogeneity in transmission that relates to patterns of mixing between groups. These analyses indicate that few disease transmission processes in the real world can be adequately described using homogeneous mixing models. Populations tend to be poorly mixed, with most individuals interacting with only a relatively small proportion of individuals within the larger population. Studies of the transmission of many diseases highlight the increased probability of transmission between members of the same family (Brimblecombe et al., 1958; Hendley et al., 1969; Hope Simpson, 1952; Monto, 1968), which is hardly surprising given the amount of time they spend in close proximity. Similarly, schoolchildren have an increased chance of acquiring infection from other children within their classroom (Fine and Clarkson, 1982; London and Yorke, 1973), as might colleagues who work together in an office (Gwaltney Jr. et al., 1966; Lidwell and Williams,

1961). On a larger scale, transmission of disease tends to be localized in space, as most individuals spend a fair part of their time close to home, visiting distant cities only infrequently. That disease transmission occurs at many different levels suggests that a hierarchical description of populations might be appropriate in many contexts, particularly in models of geographic spread.

In addition to these structural heterogeneities related to the nature of the contact process, behavioral heterogeneities resulting from activities with different associated risks have a major impact upon the spread of many diseases. They are especially important in the spread of sexually transmitted diseases (STDs), for which infection is often concentrated in high-risk groups, such as those who have a large number of partners or indulge in risky sexual behavior (May and Anderson, 1988; Yorke et al., 1978). Genetic and immunological factors can also be important. For example, possession of certain HLA alleles can be protective against or can predispose people to certain infections (Hill et al., 1991; Jeffery et al., 1999), and immune status can clearly affect the ability to overcome infection.

2.4.5.1 Heterogeneity in population-level frameworks

Within a population-level modeling framework, heterogeneity can be accounted for by refining the set of states describing members of a population, adding, for instance, descriptions of the individual's age, family, community, or genetic makeup. Notice that this can cause a substantial increase in the dimensionality of the model. If the heterogeneity involves m different groups (e.g., age classes), the number of variables appearing in the model increases by a factor of m.

The inclusion of heterogeneity also requires a description of the disease transmission process between individuals in different groups, often dubbed "who acquires infection from whom" (WAIFW). This quickly becomes a complex task — if the heterogeneity involves m different groups (e.g., age classes), one must describe $m \times m$ possible transmission terms. Although some symmetry is often assumed in this structure (such as there being an identical chance of transmission between an infectious individual in group i and a susceptible in group j as between an infectious individual in group j and a susceptible in group i), a large number of additional parameters are usually introduced.

If many different sources of heterogeneity are accounted for, it is possible for the number of groups to become comparable to the size of the population. In such cases, the complexity of the population-based description approaches that of an individual-based description, and so the latter may become a preferable alternative.

A large body of literature dealing with the formulation and epidemiological implications of different mixing patterns has been developed (e.g., Adler, 1992; Barbour, 1978; Blythe and Castillo-Chavez, 1989; Blythe et al., 1991; Busenberg and Castillo-Chavez, 1991; Castillo-Chavez and Busenberg, 1990; Diekmann et al., 1990; Dushoff et al., 2007; Gupta et al., 1989; Hethcote et al., 1982; Hethcote and Thieme, 1985; Hethcote and Van Ark, 1987; Jacquez et al., 1988; Nold, 1980). Before presenting the full formalism of the mixing-group model, we introduce some of the basic concepts by means of a simple example.

2.4.5.2 *An example of a mixing model*

Imagine two groups of people, with 2,000 people in group A and 1,000 people in group B (see Figure 2.4 to help visualize this example). We further imagine that individuals in group B are, for some reason, more active than people in group A. More specifically, we suppose that a typical member of group B meets 50 people per day, whereas a typical member of group A meets just 15 people per day. We say that the average activity level of members of group B is $3\frac{1}{3}$ times that of members of group A.

We now look at the total numbers of contacts made each day. Since each contact involves two people, there are two ways of counting these contacts — each contact can either be counted once (since there is one physical contact) or twice (because there are two people involved in each contact). It turns out that the mixing model is more simply specified if we adopt the second way of counting contacts, so this is how we shall work.

The 2,000 individuals in group A make a total of 30,000 contacts per day, whereas the 1,000 individuals in group B make a total of 50,000 contacts per day. Overall, there are 80,000 contacts made each day. (Again, to re-emphasize, we are counting each contact twice, so the figure of 80,000 really means that there are 40,000 actual contacts.) Since three-eighths of these contacts involve people from group A and five-eighths involve people from group B, we say that the fractional activity levels of the two groups are $\frac{3}{8}$ and $\frac{5}{8}$, respectively. These fractional activity levels account for both the different sizes of the groups and their different activity levels. Notice that even though there are more people in group A, the higher activity level of group B individuals means that they are responsible for making more of the contacts in the population.

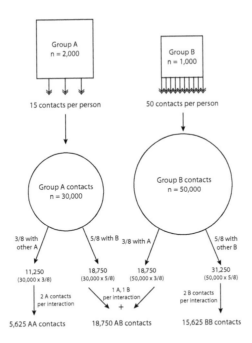

Figure 2.4 Diagram of the mixing example discussed in the text.

The final component of the mixing model is the description of how the contacts of each group are distributed between the groups: what fractions of the contacts are made with individuals of the same group and with individuals of the other group? Proportionate mixing assumes that each individual, regardless of the group he or she is in, chooses contacts randomly from the total pool of available contacts. In our example, this means that $\frac{3}{8}$ of contacts will be made with individuals in group A and $\frac{5}{8}$ of contacts will be made with individuals in group B.

What does this mean for the two groups? For group A, 11,250 contacts are made with other individuals from group A per day, whereas 18,750 contacts per day are made with individuals from group B. For group B, 18,750 contacts are made each day with individuals in group A, and 31,250 contacts per day are made with people in group B. The numbers of between-group contacts are equal, as must be the case since such contacts involve one member of group A and one member of group B.

Each within-group contact is counted twice in this calculation. In terms of actual contacts, there are 5,625 daily contacts between two

individuals who are both from group A, 15,625 daily contacts between two individuals from group B, and 18,750 daily contacts between members of different groups.

This mixing example illustrates the way in which the population
mixes, but what are the implications of mixing for an infection process? Note that in populations with heterogeneous contact patterns,
people differ in the number of contacts they make and, in addition,
these contacts are often not chosen at random from the population.
Heterogeneity in the number of contacts has a clear impact on transmission. More active susceptibles with higher numbers of contacts
meet more people, including a higher number of infectious individuals, and thus are more likely to acquire infection; similarly, more active
infectious individuals are more likely to transmit the pathogen. Notice
that the situation where individuals differ in susceptibility and/or infectivity affects only the chance of acquiring or transmitting infection,
but heterogeneity in activity affects both acquisition and transmission
of infection.

2.4.5.3 General description of mixing patterns

Mixing patterns other than proportionate mixing have been described,
and several of these are discussed below. Before moving on to these
specific models, however, we describe a general mixing model. In
order to fully understand the general model, we must first introduce
some notation. We follow the notation of Nold (1980) for the most
part; see also Hethcote and Van Ark (1987).

Let N_i be the number of individuals in the ith group. The effective
contact rate, α_{ij}, is defined as the average rate at which infectious
individuals in the jth group make effective contacts with individuals in
the ith group. This rate is the product of the rate at which individuals
in the two groups make contact and the probability, p_{ij}, that such a
contact would, if the individual in the jth group were susceptible,
lead to a disease transmission.[3] Notice that, in this formulation, it is
usually assumed that the mixing pattern is independent of the disease
statuses of individuals. In addition, it is often, although not always,
assumed that the transmission probability is symmetric: $p_{ij} = p_{ji}$.

The activity level of a group, defined as the average number of
contacts made by an individual in the given group per unit time, is
written as a_i. The mixing matrix, $\mathbf{M}$, is defined to have entries m_{ij},

---

[3]We remark that Nold employs the notation λ_{ij} for the effective contact rate,
but since we have already used λ to stand for the force of infection, we make this
minor notational change.

which give the fractions of those contacts made by an infectious individual in group j that are with individuals in group i. For example, the mixing matrix in our example above would have the form

$$\left(\begin{array}{cc} 3/8 & 3/8 \\ 5/8 & 5/8 \end{array} \right).$$

Since the entries of this matrix are fractions, the sum of the entries in any column of $\mathbf{M}$ must equal one. The contact rate between groups is therefore given by $a_j m_{ij}$, and the effective contact rate, α_{ij}, by $a_j m_{ij} p_{ij}$. It is useful to define the fractional activity levels of each group, b_i, as follows: $b_i = a_i N_i / D$. Here D is the average contact rate of the whole population, and equals the sum $\sum_i a_i N_i$. By definition, the b_i sum to one.

The mixing matrix and activity levels are subject to a set of constraints, sometimes known as balance conditions, because the number of contacts made by individuals in group i with individuals in group j must equal the number made by individuals in group j with those in group i. Hence, we have that $a_j m_{ij} N_j = a_i m_{ji} N_i$. We saw a simple illustration of such a balance condition in the example above.

We denote the average number of effective contacts made by an infectious individual in the jth group with individuals in the ith group over the course of their infectious period by t_{ij}. Together, the t_{ij} form the transmission matrix, $\mathbf{T}$. We have that $t_{ij} = \alpha_{ij} \tau_j$, where τ_j is the average duration of infection for an individual in the jth group. The effective contact number of a group, k_j, is defined to be the average number of effective contacts made by an individual in the jth group over the course of his or her infectious period, and so equals $\sum_i t_{ij}$.

2.4.5.4 Separable, proportionate, assortative, and disassortative mixing patterns

A separable mixing pattern is one for which the entries, t_{ij}, of the transmission matrix, $\mathbf{T}$, can be written as $t_{ij} = x_i y_j$. In such instances, the probability of transmission is influenced separately by the two types of individuals involved. It turns out that many analyses are particularly simple to carry out when the transmission matrix is of this form (see, for example, Diekmann and Heesterbeek, 2000, p. 223).

The proportionate mixing model, introduced by Barbour (1978) and Nold (1980) (see also Hethcote and Van Ark (1987)), assumes individuals have no preference for those with whom they interact. In other words, the chance that a given contact will be with an individual of type i is determined simply by the fractional activity level of individuals of type i. This mixing pattern is described by $m_{ij} = b_i$, which gives a matrix of the type

$$
\begin{pmatrix}
b_1 & b_1 & b_1 & b_1 \\
b_2 & b_2 & b_2 & b_2 \\
b_3 & b_3 & b_3 & b_3 \\
b_4 & b_4 & b_4 & b_4
\end{pmatrix}.
$$

Proportionate mixing is sometimes referred to as random mixing and is a special case of separable mixing.

Assortative mixing implies that groups have a higher within-group contact rate than would be expected by chance (i.e., under proportionate mixing). In this case, individuals are more likely to interact with others who are similar to them. As an example, the following matrix shows a 4x4 example in which a small amount is added to each diagonal element and one-third of that amount is subtracted from each nondiagonal element in a particular column:

$$
\begin{pmatrix}
b_1 + e & b_1 - f/3 & b_1 - g/3 & b_1 - h/3 \\
b_2 - e/3 & b_2 + f & b_2 - g/3 & b_2 - h/3 \\
b_3 - e/3 & b_3 - f/3 & b_3 + g & b_3 - h/3 \\
b_4 - e/3 & b_4 - f/3 & b_4 - g/3 & b_4 + h
\end{pmatrix}.
$$

In general, the amounts subtracted from nondiagonal elements in a particular column need not be equal to each other, but the sum of those elements must be equal to the amount added to the diagonal element in that column. Mixing that is completely assortative (i.e., mixing that occurs only with members of an individual's own group) is referred to as restricted mixing (Jacquez et al., 1988; Nold, 1980). Restricted mixing would be represented by the identity matrix (i.e., all diagonal elements are equal to 1 and all nondiagonal elements are equal to 0).

Disassortative mixing describes the situation in which within-group contact rates are lower than expected under proportionate mixing: individuals have a tendency to interact with others who are dissimilar to them. Mixing of this type would result in a matrix like that shown above for assortative mixing, although the additional amounts would be subtracted from the diagonal elements and added to the nondiagonal elements.

A commonly used example of assortative mixing is preferred mixing (Andreasen and Christiansen, 1989; Blythe and Castillo-Chavez,

1989; Hethcote et al., 1982; Hethcote and Van Ark, 1987; Hyman and Stanley, 1988; Jacquez et al., 1988; Nold, 1980), in which mixing is described by a linear combination of proportionate mixing and restricted mixing. In this situation a certain fraction of the contacts, r_i, of each group are within-group interactions, while the remaining contacts are subject to proportionate mixing. A 4x4 example of such a mixing strategy is given by the following:

$$
\begin{pmatrix}
r_1 + \frac{1-r_1}{4} & \frac{1-r_2}{4} & \frac{1-r_3}{4} & \frac{1-r_4}{4} \\
\frac{1-r_1}{4} & r_2 + \frac{1-r_2}{4} & \frac{1-r_3}{4} & \frac{1-r_4}{4} \\
\frac{1-r_1}{4} & \frac{1-r_2}{4} & r_3 + \frac{1-r_3}{4} & \frac{1-r_4}{4} \\
\frac{1-r_1}{4} & \frac{1-r_2}{4} & \frac{1-r_3}{4} & r_4 + \frac{1-r_4}{4}
\end{pmatrix}.
$$

The simplest form of preferred mixing assumes that the fraction of contacts reserved for within-group interactions (r_i) is equal across groups. The matrix above shows a more general form that varies the fraction of within-group contacts but assumes that the four groups are the same size and that their fractional activity levels are all equal. In its most general form, preferred mixing (for an SIR model) is given by

$$
r_{jj} = r_j + (1 - r_j) \frac{a_j (1 - r_j) N_j}{\sum_k a_k (1 - r_k) N_k} \tag{2.18}
$$

and

$$
r_{ij} = (1 - r_j) \frac{a_i (1 - r_j) N_i}{\sum_k a_k (1 - r_k) N_k}, \qquad j \neq i. \tag{2.19}
$$

N_k is the population size of group k, a_j is the average number of contacts made by an individual in group j per unit time, r_{jj} gives the fraction of contacts an individual from group j makes with other individuals from group j, and r_{ij} gives the fraction of contacts an individual from group j makes with individuals from group i (Jacquez et al., 1988).

2.4.5.5 Heterogeneity in individual-based frameworks

Heterogeneities in mixing patterns can also be incorporated into individual-based modeling frameworks. A natural way of describing the interactions, and hence the potential for disease transmission, between members of the population is as a graph. Individuals are represented by nodes of the graph and possible interactions between individuals

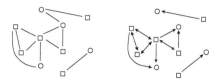

Figure 2.5 Examples of networks linking individuals within a population. The graph on the left is an undirected graph indicating when an interaction occurs between pairs of individuals. The graph on the right is a directed graph of the same network, but represents the potential transmission patterns of a theoretical disease that can only be transmitted to others by males (squares correspond to males, circles to females). Weights could be assigned to this graph if the rate of transmission between two males was different from the rate of transmission from male to female.

by edges linking nodes (Figure 2.5). A notable use of this description is within the context of sexually transmitted diseases, when the edges of the graphs represent sexual partnerships (see, for example, Klovdahl, 1985; Kretzschmar and Morris, 1996; Morris and Kretzschmar, 1995, 1997). For situations in which disease transmission is a symmetric process, i.e., the probability of transmission between a given pair of individuals is the same regardless of which of them is the susceptible and which the infectious individual, an undirected graph can be employed. In asymmetric cases, such as a sexually transmitted disease for which the male to female and female to male transmission rates differ, a directed graph must be used to indicate which type of transmission goes with which rate.

Heterogeneity in transmission can be accounted for by assigning strengths to the edges of the graph. These strengths can vary, reflecting the differing susceptibilities, infectivities, and contact patterns between different individuals that together determine the probabilities of transmission between pairs of individuals.

The graph depicting population interactions need not be constant over time. For instance, sexual partnerships change over time, so the graph structure underlying the transmission of sexually transmitted diseases has a dynamic nature.

2.4.6 Seasonal variations in transmission

Transmission risks within and among groups can vary because transmission rates may vary over time. Transmission may, for example, have a seasonal component that reflects changing climatic conditions. Behavioral changes can introduce seasonal variations, most notably in regard to those diseases for which schools are centers for disease trans- mission. In such cases, transmission rates are higher during school terms compared to vacations because students interact more closely with one another when confined within classrooms (Fine and Clark- son, 1982; London and Yorke, 1973). A number of population-based models have incorporated some kind of school scheduling in models for the spread of measles and other childhood infections (e.g., Bauch and Earn, 2003; Earn et al., 2000b; Schenzle, 1984; Stone et al., 2007). In the individual-based framework, seasonality leads to the interac- tion graph having a dynamic component, reflecting the different inter- action patterns between school terms and vacations (Keeling et al., 1997). Similar effects clearly play a role in diseases that are trans- mitted by a vector species, such as a mosquito, whose numbers vary seasonally (Aron and May, 1982).

2.5   THE BASIC REPRODUCTIVE NUMBER REVISITED

Because of the important role the basic reproductive number has played in understanding and predicting epidemic behaviors, the con- cept has been generalized to account for heterogeneity and more com- plex descriptions of the infection process. In general situations, the analysis of Diekmann et al. (1990) shows that R_0 is given by the max- imum eigenvalue of the next generation operator. This operator, in models with a discrete set of disease states, is the transmission ma- trix, $\mathbf{T}$, described earlier, whose entries give the average number of effective contacts made by an infectious individual in the jth group with individuals in the ith group over the course of the individual's infectious period.

In simple situations, the maximum eigenvalue is equal to the average number of secondary infections — the simple average, as in Equation 2.7. More generally, care must be taken when interpreting the word "average" that is often used in verbal definitions of R_0. A particularly interesting, and illuminating, example of the potential problems with loose definitions of "average" is provided by a model for a sexually transmitted disease in a heterosexual population (Diekmann et al., 1990). Neglecting behavioral heterogeneity, such a model has two effective contact numbers: one for male to female transmission, t_{12}, and the other for female to male transmission, t_{21}. In this case, the basic reproductive number is given by the geometric mean of these contact numbers: $R_0 = \sqrt{t_{12}t_{21}}$. This can be understood without resorting to the eigenvalue definition: the effective contact number of the two-step process of male to male (or female to female) transmission is given by the product $t_{12}t_{21}$. Consequently, the corresponding one-step "average" contact number must be the square root of this quantity. Notice that, as the geometric mean is always smaller than the arithmetic mean (unless the two quantities are equal, in which case the two means are equal), the (incorrect) naive definition of R_0 (involving the arithmetic mean of contact numbers) would tend to overestimate the true value.

In general, it is difficult to obtain a simple closed expression for the basic reproductive number in a heterogeneous transmission setting. One important special case in which this is possible, however, is under separable transmission, for which $t_{ij} = x_i y_j$. The important property exhibited by a transmission matrix of this type is that it has only one nonzero eigenvalue, which equals $\sum_i x_i y_i$ (Busenberg and Castillo-Chavez, 1991; Castillo-Chavez and Busenberg, 1990; Diekmann and Heesterbeek, 2000). Hence, R_0 is given by the simple expression $\sum_i x_i y_i$.

In the proportionate mixing setting, which we recall is a specific example of separable mixing, the expression for R_0 can be further simplified, and can be written in terms of the mean and variance of the contact distribution. Recalling that k_j is defined to be the average effective contact number for an individual in group j, and defining $K = \sum_j b_j k_j$, as the average of the k_j, weighted with respect to the activity levels of the groups, then

$$R_0 = K + \frac{\text{var } k}{K}$$
$$= K(1 + CV^2). \tag{2.20}$$

Here, $\text{var } k$ is the variance of the k_j and CV is their coefficient of variation (i.e., standard deviation divided by the average). A result of the form (2.20) appears in many contexts within the literature and has been rediscovered on numerous occasions (Anderson et al., 1986; Barbour, 1978; Dietz, 1980; Dye and Hasibeder, 1986; May and Anderson, 1988). Hethcote and Van Ark (1987) give an equivalent expression, although they do not mention that it can be expressed in terms of the variance.

The important point to notice about Equation 2.20 is that the variance of the distribution makes an additional contribution to the value of R_0. In other words, heterogeneity tends to increase the value of R_0. This result can be traced back to the earlier comment that highly active individuals contribute disproportionately to transmission: their high activity level means that they are more likely to acquire infection and also more likely to transmit infection. In situations where there is significant heterogeneity, use of models that assume perfect mixing can be misleading in important ways. For instance, even if the mean effective contact number lies below one, R_0 can still be greater than one because of the variability in the contact distribution.

Equation 2.20 is a particular example of a slightly more general result, obtained in a situation in which the groups differ in their susceptibilities, which we denote by A_i, and their infectiousnesses, denoted by B_i. In a fairly general model, it can be shown (Becker and Marschner, 1990; Woolhouse et al., 1998) that the basic reproductive number for the heterogeneous model is obtained by multiplying that of the corresponding homogeneous model (i.e., the model in which the average of the A_i and the average of the B_i are employed) by a factor of the form

$$1 + CV(A)CV(B)\rho(A, B), \qquad (2.21)$$

where $CV(A)$ and $CV(B)$ are the coefficients of variation of the A_i and the B_i, and $\rho(A, B)$ is the correlation coefficient between them. Notice that if the susceptibilities and infectiousnesses are proportional to each other, the correlation coefficient is equal to one and the two coefficients of variation will be equal. This is the case in our mixing group example since both factors arise from the differing activity levels. The resulting factor is simply that given by Equation 2.20.

Explicit expressions for R_0 are, for general mixing patterns, difficult to find. In some cases, such as the preferred mixing pattern discussed above, a limited analysis shows that R_0 must satisfy a particular simple nonlinear equation. From this equation, a threshold condition for an epidemic can be deduced (Andreasen and Christiansen, 1989; Blythe and Castillo-Chavez, 1989; Diekmann et al., 1990; Diekmann and Heesterbeek, 2000).

2.5.1 Implications of heterogeneity for disease transmission and control

As we have seen, in heterogeneous settings, highly active individuals often contribute disproportionately to transmission. For many sexually transmitted diseases, the average contact number (taken over the whole population, and without weighting by the activity level of different individuals) is less than one, and yet the disease does not go extinct. The circulation of such diseases may be maintained by a relatively small group of highly sexually active individuals, such as sex workers or a highly promiscuous group of people. Such highly active groups of individuals are known as core groups for the infection (Yorke et al., 1978). The disease prevalence within a core group is high, while the prevalence in the population at large is low, with the result that the core groups account for a large proportion of cases within the overall population.

Analysis of models that incorporate these mixing patterns into the standard compartmental modeling framework show that the nature of mixing assumptions can significantly affect the timing and rate of spread of diseases through the groups, as well as the total severity of the epidemic (see, for example, Gupta et al., 1989; Jacquez et al., 1988; Kaplan, 1989; Morris, 1993; Sattenspiel and Dietz, 1995; Sattenspiel and Herring, 1998; Sattenspiel et al., 2000).

Heterogeneity in transmission has important implications for the control of disease, most notably in those situations that exhibit the core group phenomenon. Since the prevalence in the noncore group is low, treatment or vaccination of that group has relatively little effect. Control measures applied to the core group, on the other hand, can have a dramatic effect, rapidly decreasing transmission. In heterogeneous situations, control policies must account for the heterogeneity — uniform control policies will be much less effective than in a well-mixed case, whereas targeted control will be most effective.

2.5.2 Estimation of the basic reproductive number

Given the importance of the basic reproductive number, many studies in mathematical epidemiology have sought to estimate its value in real-world situations (see, for example, Anderson, 1982; Anderson et al., 1988; Gani and Leach, 2001). Despite its simplicity, both in terms of its verbal definition and its expression in terms of model parameters, the measurement of R_0 is often far from simple. Parameters such as the transmission parameter, β, are difficult to measure directly. As a consequence, estimation of R_0 usually proceeds in an indirect fashion, most often via the relationships expressed in Equations 2.8, 2.9, or 2.13, which relate R_0 to more easily observed properties of the system, such as the initial growth rate of an epidemic, the susceptible fraction at equilibrium, or the size of an epidemic observed in a closed population.

It is important to understand, however, that such relationships are model dependent. In more complex model settings, the relationship between R_0 and the observable quantity might be quite different, and so estimates of R_0 obtained in this way must be treated with caution. For instance, estimates based on the relationship relating R_0 to the initial exponential rate of increase of the number of infectious individuals are highly dependent on the description of the infection time course employed by the model. As an example, Nowak et al. (1997) attempted to estimate R_0 for a within-host situation (cell to cell transmission of SIV within an individual monkey) and found that, in their case, estimates could vary by an order of magnitude, depending on the assumptions made in their model (see also Lloyd, 2001b).

Another point that needs to be borne in mind when dealing with numerical estimates of R_0 is that this quantity is a property both of the disease and of the host population under consideration. The value of R_0 governing a disease process in one population setting need not equal its value in another situation. This cautions against the uncritical use of an R_0 value measured in a given population setting for predicting epidemic properties in other situations.

The concepts discussed in this chapter include many of the issues that need to be considered when developing any type of mathematical model for infectious disease transmission. In our next chapter we focus on how mathematical epidemiologists have studied the geographic spread of influenza epidemics in particular. The examples described will highlight the kinds of questions addressed in geographic models and the types of results and insights derived from the use of epidemic models in a geographic framework. They are intended to provide a context that will result in better understanding of the specific strategies used to model geographic spread — the details of which we will begin to discuss in Chapter 4.

Chapter Three

Modeling the Geographic Spread of
Influenza Epidemics

Some of the earliest models describing the geographic spread of infectious diseases were developed to understand and predict the spread of influenza epidemics, and such models continue to provide the foundation for important present-day research. Most early models for the geographic spread of influenza epidemics as well as several more recent models have approached the problem from the perspective of the population. In other words, these models assume that all individuals within a population or its subgroups can be treated equally. In recent years, however, and in response to the growing fear of a new world-wide influenza pandemic, individual-based models have been developed and applied towards understanding how influenza spreads within and across populations and how its spread might be minimized if a new strain enters the human population. In this chapter we illustrate the kinds of questions that both population-based and individual-based models have addressed, and we compare and contrast the advantages and disadvantages of each of these approaches, both for understanding the spread of influenza epidemics and for modeling the geographic spread of other infectious diseases.

3.1 A BRIEF OVERVIEW OF THE BIOLOGY OF INFLUENZA

Naturally occurring influenza epidemics have been a fact of human life for centuries, and they have often resulted in high rates of mortality. For example, the number of world-wide deaths during the 1918-19 epidemic has recently been estimated to be at least 50 million, with an average world-wide mortality rate of about 5 deaths per thousand people (Johnson and Mueller, 2002). Influenza epidemics have also seriously disrupted social and economic relations among populations and communities (Glezen, 1996). The impact of the disease is not limited to world-wide pandemics, however. The United States alone experiences over 35,000 influenza-related deaths annually. The impact

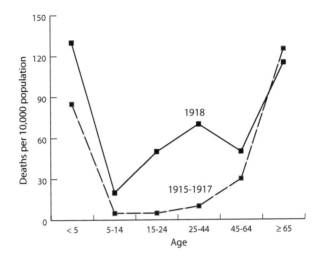

Figure 3.1 The age distribution of influenza deaths before and during the 1918-19
influenza epidemic. Notice the U-shaped pattern of 1915-17 and the
contrasting W-shaped pattern of 1918. Data taken from Olson et al.
(2005), Figure 2a.

during normal years is especially high for the oldest and youngest individuals, leading to a U-shaped age-specific mortality curve (Figure
3.1). Furthermore, the numbers of deaths in the United States have
increased over the last quarter century (Simonsen et al., 1998; Thompson et al., 2003). Although the impact of the disease is usually highest
for the very young and the very old, unusual epidemics, such as the
1918-19 pandemic, have been known to differentially affect individuals at the prime of life. This epidemic signature of high mortality at
intermediate ages leads to a W-shaped mortality pattern rather than
the normal U-shaped pattern (Figure 3.1).

One of the characteristic features of the influenza virus is its ability
to quickly and regularly evolve into new strains (Palese, 1993). The
virus has two surface antigens: hemagglutinin, which is used to bind
the virus to the host cell and initiate reproduction, and neuraminidase,
which aids in the release from host cells of newly manufactured viral particles and thus aids viral spread. Evolutionary changes in the
virus can occur through antigenic "drift," caused by simple mutations that lead to minor changes in the surface proteins (most often
the hemagglutinin), through antigenic "shift," a major change in the

surface proteins that essentially results in a new form of the virus to which most individuals are not immune, and occasionally through the direct introduction of an animal strain of influenza into the human population (Kaplan and Webster, 1977; Scholtissek, 1994). The latter situation generally results in severe disease but limited transmission to other humans (Hilleman, 2002) and appears to be the present status of avian influenza in Asia.

Antigenic drift is a consequence of constant, usually minor mutations in the viral RNA. The accumulation of these mutations eventually results in a virus that has changed enough that it cannot be fought off by the immune system of individuals previously exposed to earlier forms of the virus. In any one year, however, only a minority of individuals in a population will lack sufficient immunity to the circulating strain to become infected. This kind of mechanism causes the relatively mild yearly outbreaks that are characteristic of influenza.

Antigenic shifts in the structure of the virus have a more severe impact on the human host and underlie the three major 20th-century pandemics — the 1918-19 Spanish flu pandemic, the 1957-58 Asian flu pandemic, and the 1968-69 Hong Kong flu pandemic. Antigenic shifts usually occur as a consequence of reassortment of genetic material from different influenza strains, which may be derived from multiple species besides humans (most commonly birds, but occasionally other species, especially swine) (Hilleman, 2002; Reid et al., 2004; Taubenberger and Morens, 2006b). These structural changes usually result in viruses with a completely or largely new antigenic structure. Consequently, the vast majority of individuals do not possess underlying immunity and are thus susceptible to infection.

In addition to its capacity for rapid evolutionary change, the influenza virus is moderately infectious and can be transmitted readily from one person to another. The disease progression within an individual is shown in Figure 3.2. Transmission occurs through airborne spread in droplets derived from the coughs and sneezes of an infectious person and by direct droplet contact (Heymann, 2004). The disease can be very difficult to control since active transmission can begin within one day after infection, before a person is totally aware of being sick. Once symptoms appear, a person generally remains infectious for 3-5 more days. Recovery from a true case of influenza occurs after about one week and leads to the development of immunity to the particular strain causing the infection and closely related strains (Heymann, 2004). However, because of the rapid evolution of the virus, individuals remain susceptible to infection with new strains of the virus. This lack of immunity to new strains and the ease of

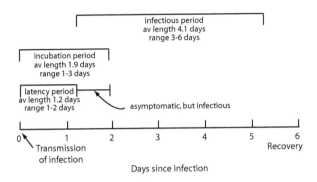

Figure 3.2 The progression of an influenza infection.

transmission of the virus have resulted in repeated world-wide epidemics, with broad patterns of spread across time and space that are well recognized. This has stimulated several attempts to develop mathematical models that would predict these patterns and so help to prevent future world-wide pandemics.

3.2 POPULATION-BASED INFLUENZA MODELS

3.2.1 Model structures and general results

The majority of models for the geographic spread of influenza are population-based models (and specifically metapopulation models; see Chapter 4). The models generally divide the population of interest into subgroups determined by disease status, community, risk group, and other factors deemed important, and variation among individuals within a given subgroup is ignored. In addition, the models only account for changes in the numbers of people in each group, rather than the fates of specific individuals.

Almost all of the population-based influenza models are applications of an influential model originally developed in the mid- to late 1960s by O.V. Baroyan, L.A. Rvachev, and colleagues in the former Soviet Union (Baroyan and Rvachev, 1967; Baroyan et al., 1969, 1971; Baroyan and Rvachev, 1978) (referred to in the following as the BR model). This model was developed further by Rvachev and Longini (1985) and Longini (1988). Studies using this model have included both models for forecasting influenza epidemics within a single city or region (e.g., Aguirre and Gonzalez, 1992) and models focused on either forecasting influenza epidemics across multiple cities or regions or reproducing past patterns to explore the feasibility of forecasting future epidemics (e.g., the Russian work of Baroyan and colleagues, Flahault et al., 1988, 1994; Grais et al., 2003, 2004; Hyman and LaForce, 2003; Spicer, 1979). In addition, Flahault et al. (2006) recently used the BR model and Cooper et al. (2006) used a stochastic analog of the model to test the impact of potential interventions on the spread of an influenza pandemic.

The formulation of the BR model used most often is a deterministic discrete time SEIR (susceptible/exposed/infectious/recovered) model in a continuous state space. It is based on an interacting system of n cities that are linked to each other by means of a transportation network. Empirically derived probability distributions are used to model the length of the latent period and the length of the infectious period. The model also keeps track of the number of individuals who become infectious on day t (the daily incidence) and the number of newly reported cases.

Within each city, individuals are assumed to mix homogeneously. Individuals may also travel from one city to another according to a transportation operator. In early models the transportation matrix was assumed to be symmetric — the number of passengers traveling from city i to city j was set equal to the number of passengers traveling from city j to city i; this assumption was relaxed in Longini (1988), although applications of the model often retain the assumption due to the reduction in the amount of data required for a symmetric model.

In the equations below we use the formulation of Rvachev and Longini (1985), with minor changes. Rvachev and Longini (1985) and also Grais et al. (2003) may be consulted for more complete details on the structure of the model. For each community, i, let $S_i(t)$ be the number of susceptibles at time t, $E_i(\tau, t)$ be the number of exposed individuals at time t who were infected at time $t - \tau$, $I_i(\tau, t)$ be the number of infectious individuals at time t who were infected τ time units earlier, and $R_i(t)$ be the number of recovered individuals at time t. Let τ_1 and τ_2 be the maximum lengths of the latent and infectious periods, respectively. The total population size is assumed constant so that

$$S_i(t) + \sum_{\tau=0}^{\tau_1} E_i(\tau, t) + \sum_{\tau=0}^{\tau_2} I_i(\tau, t) + R_i(t) = N_i \qquad \text{for every } t. \quad (3.1)$$

The transportation operator used in this model was designed to operate on any dynamic variable $A_i(t)$ and takes the form

$$\Omega[A_i(t)] = A_i(t) + \sum_{j=1}^{n} \left[A_j(t)\frac{\sigma_{ji}}{N_j} - A_i(t)\frac{\sigma_{ij}}{N_i} \right], \qquad (3.2)$$

where σ_{ij} is the daily passenger flow from community i to community j. This transportation operator is used to govern the movement of noninfectious individuals; infectious individuals are assumed not to travel. In addition, the daily infectious contact rate, or the average number of individuals with whom an infectious person will make contact sufficient to transmit infection, is denoted as λ.

The full model consists of a system of difference equations for a group of n communities. The equations for each community i take the following forms:

$$S_i(t+1) = \Omega[S_i(t)] - E_i(0,t) \qquad (3.3)$$

$$E_i(\tau+1, t+1) = (1 - \gamma(\tau))\Omega[E_i(\tau,t)] \quad \text{if } \tau = 0, 1, \ldots, \tau_1 - 1 \quad (3.4)$$

$$I_i(\tau+1, t+1) = \begin{cases} \gamma(\tau)\Omega[E_i(\tau,t)] + (1 - \delta(\tau))I_i(\tau,t) \\ \qquad \text{if } \tau = 0, 1, \ldots, \tau_1 \\ (1 - \delta(\tau))I_i(\tau,t) \\ \qquad \text{if } \tau = \tau_1 + 1, \tau_1 + 2, \ldots, \tau_2 - 1 \end{cases} \qquad (3.5)$$

$$R_i(t+1) = \sum_{\tau=0}^{\tau_1} \gamma(\tau)\Omega[E_i(\tau,t)], \qquad (3.6)$$

where $\gamma(\tau)$ is the probability that an exposed individual becomes infectious on day $\tau + 1$ given that the individual was still in the latent stage on day τ and $\delta(\tau)$ is the probability that an infectious individual recovers on day $\tau + 1$ given that the individual was still infectious on day τ. In real populations only a fraction of influenza cases are reported to the authorities and these are the data actually available to compare to the model. Consequently, both Rvachev and Longini (1985) and Grais et al. (2003) estimated reported cases by multiplying the total number of cases (given by Equation 3.6) by a reporting rate, which did not vary among communities.

The boundary conditions for the model are given by

$$E_i(0, t) = S_i(t) \frac{\lambda}{N_i} \sum_{\tau=1}^{\tau_2} E_i(0, t - \tau) g(\tau) \qquad (3.7)$$

and

$$I_i(0, t) = 0. \qquad (3.8)$$

$g(\tau)$ is the fraction of individuals who were initially infected at the same time and are in the infectious state at time τ. Equation 3.7 gives the number of newly exposed individuals who are infected by infectious individuals in city i on day t.

In order to test the model, Baroyan et al. (1969) used data from a 1965 influenza epidemic and modeled the spread of the disease among the 128 largest cities in the USSR. Initially they were not able to get adequate transportation data, so they assumed that the strength of interaction between two cities was proportional to the product of their population size. The proportionality constant was chosen to give a satisfactory fit to observed data. Estimates of other parameters were derived from epidemiological data collected during the epidemic. Serological surveys did not provide data sufficient to estimate the number of susceptibles at the start of the epidemic — the proportion of influenza cases among all acute respiratory infections could not be detected and even when surveys were conducted during epidemics the percentage of positive identifications of the virus was very small. Consequently, the initial numbers of susceptibles used in numerical simulations of the model were based on the number of cases in the city where the outbreak was first registered. Baroyan et al. (1969) assumed that this city was representative of all other cities and used its estimated initial proportion of susceptibles (40% of the initial population) for all cities.

It is important to realize that these assumptions were made in the context of modeling nonpandemic influenza scenarios, and so they reflect quite strong views about a "normal" situation for which there is little accurate information. Many of the models to be discussed later in this section focus on the introduction of new strains into a population, and the consequent potential for pandemic spread. This disease invasion setting is much easier to deal with than the relatively endemic situation modeled by Baroyan and colleagues, because in the pandemic situation it is assumed that all individuals are susceptible except for the index case.

A simulated epidemic was run from 4 January to 1 March 1965.

Outbreaks developed in all towns, with the simulated outbreaks occurring about 2-3 weeks prior to onset of the real outbreak in corresponding towns. In Moscow, the simulated epidemic onset deviated from the real epidemic onset by only one day, did not last quite as long as the actual epidemic, peaked on the same day, and deviated in total number of cases and peak number of cases by about 10%. Initially, actual influenza epidemic data for the other cities were not recorded at an appropriate time interval to allow the detailed comparisons available for Moscow. However, such data became available in 1970, allowing case numbers in real epidemics and simulated epidemics in a number of cities to be compared (Baroyan et al., 1970). Expected numbers resulting from model simulations were sometimes very close to the observed number of cases, but were sometimes quite different (see Figure 3.3 for examples).

It is likely that the earlier onset of the epidemic in simulated outbreaks (which is also seen in other studies using the BR model) is partly or largely a consequence of the population-based and deterministic formulation of the model. In formulations such as that used in the BR model fractional individuals can spread an epidemic — the model is not constrained to whole individuals. Furthermore, epidemic transmission is certain to occur as long as there is a positive rate of transmission (i.e., there are no stochastic effects to limit spread when transmission rates and numbers of infected individuals are low, either initially or during the course of an epidemic). As these differences between deterministic, population-based models and stochastic, individual-based models are important, we will return to them periodically in later sections of the book.

Baroyan et al. (1969) also explored the effects of varying the parameter values used in the model, with the following results:

1) The incidence and maximum number of cases in a simulated city were strongly influenced by the proportion of the population initially susceptible to the disease.

2) An epidemic threshold was clearly seen in a number of the analyses, such that when the initial proportion of susceptibles was too small, an epidemic would not occur.

3) The incidence and maximum number of cases increased with increasing probability of transmission of the disease.

4) There was a logistic relationship between the intensity of passenger exchange and the time interval between onsets of epidemics

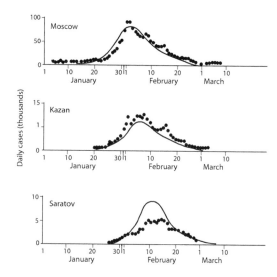

Figure 3.3 Examples of simulations of the Baroyan-Rvachev model in three Russian towns. Dots show the observed case numbers; curves are the results of simulations for each city. Adapted from Fine (1982) and Baroyan et al. (1970).

in cities and maximum morbidity times, with the epidemic onset times and maximum morbidity times occurring earlier with increasing passenger exchange until an exchange rate was reached at which they no longer changed.

The authors noted that this logistic behavior was dependent on the intensity of passenger exchange among cities being much smaller than the frequency of contacts within a city, which is almost certainly a reasonable assumption.

Baroyan and Rvachev (1978) used this model in combination with data on bus and rail transportation to forecast future cases of influenza through the mid-1970s. Unlike the earlier work of Baroyan et al. (1969) they also were able to use observed influenza data from many different cities rather than just from Moscow. The results of their predictions are as follows:

1) Using data from 1957-1970 — 80% of the time the predicted peak day was within one week of the actual peak day and 55% of the time the height of the predicted peak was within a range of deviation defined by the authors to be desirable (1.5 times

lower or higher than the actual peak).

2) 1971-72 — 90% of the time the predicted peak day was within one week of the actual peak day and 80% of the time the height of the predicted peak was within the desirable range of deviation.

3) 1973 — 96% of the time the predicted peak day was within one week of the actual peak day and 78% of the time the height of the predicted peak was within the desirable range of deviation.

Results for 1975 and 1976 were similar. Baroyan and Rvachev (1978) concluded that the predictive value of the model was satisfactory for the USSR and postulated that since a satisfactory model could be built for such a vast territory, it is likely that analogous models could be constructed for other states as long as the appropriate data were available.

As cited in Longini et al. (1986), the Russian model was later expanded to include 232 Soviet cities (Belova et al., 1982) and a similar model was applied in Bulgaria (Baroyan et al., 1978). Rvachev and Longini (1985) and Longini (1988) applied the model to the global spread of the 1968-69 Hong Kong flu epidemic and found that the model could also reproduce general space-time patterns of spread at a global level. More specifically, they found that from its start in Hong Kong, the epidemic spread throughout the northern hemisphere and then later spread to the southern hemisphere, corresponding to the 6-month lag in seasons between the two hemispheres. It is important to note, however, that this seasonal activity was built into the structure of their model — the daily infectious contact rate during the nonepidemic periods in the northern and southern hemispheres was reduced to 10% of its epidemic period value to reflect higher levels of contact present during the winter season in a particular hemisphere, while no adjustment was made in tropical regions.

Flahault et al. (1988) applied a simplified continuous-time version of the BR model to a 1984-85 influenza epidemic in twenty-two French metropolitan districts, basing their transportation operator on rail data linking the cities. Their estimates of epidemiological parameters were derived from data collected in 1984 through the French Computer Network for the Surveillance of Communicable Diseases, a compilation of illness reports from general practitioners located throughout the country.

Flahault et al. (1988) did not have certain knowledge of where the epidemic started, so in their simulations they assumed a simultaneous

onset in Nord-Pas-de-Calais and in Aquitaine, with 5 cases per physician. Their computed results did not fit the observed data in each
district, but general trends were often predicted by the model. For example, an east-west dark band (more than 10 cases per physician) was
predicted and observed at weeks 7 and 8. The actual epidemic ended
in the northeast of the country, and that was also predicted by the
model. Results from predictions at the district level were mixed, however. The model only produced unimodal curves, but some districts
experienced bimodal epidemics. In most cases with poor predictions,
the observed peak was much earlier than the simulated peak.

Flahault et al. (1994) used the same methods to simulate the spread
of influenza among 9 European cities. In this case, air transportation
data were used to estimate the degree of contact among cities. Results
indicated that an epidemic of a highly contagious disease such as
influenza was likely to spread to all cities within about one month,
implying that the time window for action by public health authorities
would be very short.

Grais et al. (2003) used the BR model with international air transportation data to predict the spread of an influenza epidemic among
the same 52 world cities modeled by Rvachev and Longini (1985) and
Longini (1988). Their goal was to determine whether and how the
general results of the earlier work would be changed with modern
rates and patterns of air travel. They also allowed the seasonal reduction in transmission in the northern and southern hemispheres to
vary monthly, although their functional relationship was not derived
from actual data on seasonal transmission; rather it was a nearly
linear relationship ranging over a 6-month period from no reduction
in transmission to the 90% reduction used by Rvachev and Longini
(1985). Simulations suggested two important potential changes. First,
a modern-day epidemic would probably spread simultaneously to both
the northern and southern hemispheres, unlike the delayed interhemi-
sphere spread predicted and observed by Rvachev and Longini (1985).
Second, as Flahault et al. (1994) suggested for European cities, Grais
et al. (2003) concluded that the global time lag for intervention would
be very short.

Grais and colleagues also used the BR model to study the spread
of influenza within the United States between 1998 and 2001 (Grais
et al., 2004). Their results were broadly similar to those of the earlier Russian work — the model generally reproduced the broad-scale
patterns observed in actual data from the influenza epidemic, but the
quality of fit to individual cities was mixed, with epidemics in some
cities predicted fairly well, but others much less adequately (each year

was considered individually in their results).

Hyman and LaForce (2003) modeled influenza epidemics in the U.S. over a 5-year period between 1996 and 2001. Their study attempted to model the normal yearly fluctuations in influenza incidence and compared the entire 5-year time series in each city to a 5-year model prediction derived from a single set of parameters. They found that their model approximated the essential features of influenza and pneumonia mortality patterns as reported by the CDC. The magnitude and fluctuations of yearly epidemics observed in the data were also reproduced by the model. In addition, in their model the number of cities included in a network and the timing of an outbreak significantly influenced the initial spread of a new infectious agent.

The most recent applications of the BR model, Flahault et al. (2006) and Cooper et al. (2006) (who used a stochastic analog), analyzed the impact of various potential interventions on the spread of an influenza pandemic. Flahault et al. (2006) considered the effect of vaccination, case isolation, therapeutic and prophylactic antiviral treatments, and air traffic reduction. Cooper et al. (2006) also looked at the effect of reducing air traffic and, in addition, they considered a general effect of reducing local transmission (which would include the joint effects of the other factors considered by Flahault et al. (2006)). They also examined the effects of seasonal variations, tropical vs. temperate environments, and several other factors. Results from both studies suggested that air traffic would have to be stopped nearly completely in order for such an intervention to have much impact — a requirement that would probably be impossible to fulfill in real situations. Both studies also found that reducing local transmission was likely to be a more efficient strategy, and, in particular, Cooper et al. (2006) suggested that isolation of cases and vaccination were likely to be the most important means of reducing local transmission.

Two other applications of the BR model deserve brief mention. Both of these papers used a local approximation presented in Baroyan et al. (1971) and Rvachev and Longini (1985). This approximation, analogous to the general Kermack-McKendrick model, considers the spread of the epidemic within one community and ignores the transportation process linking different communities. Spicer (1979) used the model to fit all influenza epidemics recorded in England and Wales between 1958 and 1973 as well as individual epidemics in greater London. He found that the fit was good and of the same order as the Russian work unless the observed epidemics were bimodal. Generally speaking, he found that the fitted curve was too high at the beginning of an epidemic and too low at the end, a result that he did not find surprising, since it is known that there is a tendency to underreport at first and then overreport at later stages of an epidemic. As discussed above in relation to the Russian work, another possible reason for this result relates to the deterministic nature of the model, since real epidemics, especially during their early stages, are highly stochastic. Aguirre and Gonzalez (1992) also used the local approximation of the BR model to forecast a 1988 influenza epidemic in Havana, Cuba. They felt that the model was sufficiently accurate to warrant its use as a practical forecasting tool in Cuba.

Stimulated by the transportation approach of Baroyan and colleagues, Sattenspiel and Dietz (1995) explicitly modeled the mobility process linking communities (i.e., the actual movement of individuals across the landscape). Their work estimated individual movement from available data and, unlike many of the other studies described above, did not assume symmetric travel patterns. The model keeps track of both the home community of travelers and of the community they are visiting. This allows it to consider who is actually present within a community at the time of contact, including regular residents and visitors from other communities (see Figure 3.4). In this model the risk of transmission is based on that group of individuals rather than the census population, which easily allows one to make the transmission risk dependent on local risk factors such as variations in sanitation, community structure, or behaviors associated with the place of contact. This model has been applied to the spread of the 1918-19 influenza epidemic in central Canadian fur trapping communities (Herring and Sattenspiel, 2003; Sattenspiel and Herring, 1998; Sattenspiel et al., 2000). Results have illustrated the relative importance of rates of mobility and within community social contact in determining timing and size of epidemic peaks. The model has also been used to address the question of whether attempts at limiting travel among communities through quarantine, as noted in the historic record, would have had any impact on the epidemic (Sattenspiel and Herring, 2003).

3.2.2 Data issues related to population-based geographic models

Applications of the population-based geographic models to pandemic situations require two primary types of data: information on cases of the disease in question and information on the amount and type of contact among individuals within and between communities or regions. In addition, in order to apply such models to nonpandemic conditions, information on the relative susceptibility of a population

a) Initial population composition and mobility structure

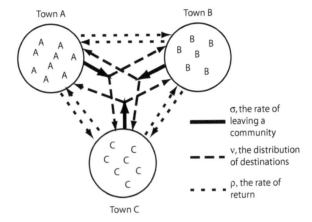

b) Composition of the towns as a consequence of the mobility

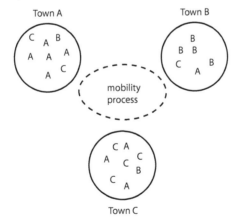

Figure 3.4 The mobility model of Sattenspiel and Dietz (1995). a) Model structure. b) Community composition as a consequence of the mobility.

is also required. The majority of the studies described above compared the results of model simulations to disease incidence data that were reported at least weekly (e.g., Flahault et al., 1988, 1994; Grais et al., 2004; Hyman and LaForce, 2003; Spicer, 1979). The Cuban study (Aguirre and Gonzalez, 1992) compared observed daily cases to daily forecasts using the local approximation of the BR model. The earliest Russian studies were able to use daily incidence data for Moscow; later studies incorporated daily incidence rates for several other cities. Incidence data for the global studies of Rvachev and Longini (1985), Longini (1988), and Grais et al. (2003) varied from city to city, ranging from daily or weekly incidence data to data on peak time and duration of the epidemic only to no incidence data at all.

In many modern-day places and in many past populations, data on the number of cases of influenza are not readily available; rather, the available data record only the numbers of deaths from the disease. As an example, the only influenza data available for the historical Canadian studies of Sattenspiel and Herring (Herring and Sattenspiel, 2003; Sattenspiel and Herring, 1998; Sattenspiel et al., 2000; Sattenspiel and Herring, 2003) were data on numbers of deaths in the communities during the epidemic. Furthermore, because of the winter timing of the epidemic and its impact on the communities, actual date of death was not always recorded, resulting in significant clumping of the data within the overall span of the epidemic. A further issue of importance with regards to influenza data is that until very recently in most places, including the United States and western Europe, either influenza and pneumonia were categorized together, or deaths were recorded under the category "influenza-like illnesses."

It is important to remember the essential time course of influenza within an individual and a population. Recent studies have estimated an average serial interval or generation time for influenza of 2.6 days (Ferguson et al., 2005). (The serial interval is the average time from infection of a single individual to the first secondary case in a contact of that individual.) With such a short generation time, a typical influenza epidemic will run its course at a particular location within a few weeks to a few months. Thus, data reported at intervals greater than weekly will not be able to capture the pattern of spread of local and regional epidemics to any extent, although studies done at the scale of large countries like Russia or the U.S. or at the global scale may be able to get by with coarser-grained data. Fortunately, in most parts of the world today, influenza is reported at least weekly during peak seasons, and many countries are beginning to set up daily surveillance networks like that which has been present in France since the mid-1980s.

Data on the amount and type of contact among individuals within and between communities and regions have also been problematic. In nearly all regions of the world today humans are highly mobile, and they use a variety of transportation modes to get from one place to another. All of the studies described above have made use of at least one source of transportation data, but in nearly every case the picture derived from analyses of the data used is at best an approximation of real patterns. For example, in their study of the 1985 influenza epidemic in France, Flahault et al. (1988) used only rail transportation data, while in their study of the spread of influenza among European cities (Flahault et al., 1994) they used only air transportation data. Grais et al. (2003, 2004), Hyman and LaForce (2003), Longini (1988), and Rvachev and Longini (1985) also used only air transportation data in their studies. Especially for studies focused at the nation level, like the French and U.S. studies of Flahault, Grais, Hyman, and their colleagues, actual travel is completed through multiple modes of transportation, including private road transportation and bus transportation as well as rail and air transportation, and these additional modes of transportation may be very important within the entire network, especially when comparing locations that are relatively close spatially. It is not clear how the picture would change if additional types of transportation data were included in these studies.

The issue of multiple modes of transportation is less important for the Russian studies, the global studies, and the Canadian studies. Both bus and air travel were included in the Russian studies, and as pointed out by Flahault et al. (1988), the Russians were able to get very good information on transportation between cities because passport control was required for all intercity travel within Russia, a situation that does not occur in most parts of the world. When looking at disease spread at the global level, the vast majority of travel, of necessity, will be air travel, which means that the air transportation network is probably a fairly good estimate of the overall network linking the cities involved. And in the Canadian studies of Sattenspiel and Herring, the environmental setting was such that the archival materials they used recorded a very high proportion of the actual travel occurring on the landscape. However, the local and special nature of this study does not easily generalize to the modern situation in most countries.

In addition to the issue of multiple modes of transportation, the major difficulties associated with transportation data relate to first obtaining such data and then to dealing with the inherent complexities and sheer volume of the data. In their initial studies, Baroyan et al. (1969) were unable to gain access to actual data and were forced to estimate exchange rates between communities by making the exchange proportional to the product of the population sizes of the communities involved. In some studies, especially earlier ones such as Rvachev and Longini (1985), the models were simplified in such a way that they used only the net exchange between two cities, rather than explicit rates of travel from A to B and from B to A. Consequently, the models assumed that the exchange rates were the same in each direction, which led to a symmetric transportation matrix. Advances in computer power are such that most more recent studies have made use of the full transportation data, although the studies generally consider a small subset of the world's cities. Additional problems related to data complexity include seasonal variation in travel rates, how to account for nondirect paths between two cities, and how to deal with trips with a total travel time that is longer than the latent period of the disease (Grais et al., 2003).

Recently, substantial effort has been devoted to elucidating complete patterns of interaction between communities, at least on a national and global scale when air travel is of overwhelming importance. Guimerà and Amaral (2004) used a database available from OAG, a global travel and transportation company, to study the nature of the world-wide travel network; Li and Cai (2004) worked with Chinese air travel data; Brownstein et al. (2006) used a United States Department of Transportation airline travel database to estimate travel patterns in the United States; and Colizza et al. (2006a,b) and Cooper et al. (2006) used the International Air Transport Association database for 2002 to estimate world-wide air travel patterns. As described above, the main purpose of the Cooper et al. study was to evaluate the impact of different interventions, while the other studies were focused more on either determining the basic structure of the air network or elucidating the relationship between air travel and regional or global patterns of influenza. This last purpose was also the aim of a recent study of spatial patterns of influenza in the United States (Viboud et al., 2006). Finally, in a very interesting and creative slant to the problem of estimating human travel patterns, Brockmann et al. (2006) used the circulation of bank notes in the United States as a proxy measure of human travel, and attempted to express these travel patterns mathematically.

Recognizing the difficulty with the availability of adequate mobility data and the problems with getting it into a manageable form,

Bonabeau et al. (1998) used spatial correlation analyses (a standard geographical technique) of data from the French Computer Network for the Surveillance of Communicable Diseases to address the question of whether geographical space, including heterogeneities in population distribution, really helps to predict more effectively the spread of an influenza epidemic. They found that for rates of travel observed in modern populations, models assuming global homogeneous (and instantaneous, within a week) geographic mixing are appropriate to describe the initial spread of an epidemic and that geographic heterogeneities and density dependence play a role only in the few weeks around an epidemic's peak. Consequently, they suggest that the question of interest be considered carefully when determining the overall complexity of the model to be used and caution that for certain kinds of questions, increasing model complexity may be neither necessary nor advisable.

3.2.3 Pluses and minuses of population-based geographic models

With rare exceptions, population-based models for the geographic spread of influenza have been used to study the spread of the disease at the large region or global scale. Models focusing on this scale, of necessity, ignore variation at smaller scales, and therefore predict only very broad patterns of spread. In at least some cases, the results of these models provide some information on the relative timing of outbreaks in different locations, and at the global scale they can perhaps provide lead time for implementing control strategies. Model results from studies at smaller scales, such as the studies in France, however, indicate that the predicted lead time would be so short that controls would not be able to be implemented in time to affect the course of an epidemic. Furthermore, simulated outbreaks tend to begin earlier than observed outbreaks, although when explicit delays are built in, as in Rvachev and Longini (1985), the models provide adequate predictions of the relative timing of outbreaks in different locations. Predictions about the magnitudes of epidemic peaks and the durations of epidemics are usually less adequate, however.

The smaller-scale work of Sattenspiel and Herring may provide some insight into this last observation. They found that varying patterns of mobility could dramatically influence the timing of epidemic peaks but had very little effect on the magnitude of the peaks (Sattenspiel and Herring, 1998). Their conclusion was that travel among communities was crucial for introducing a disease into a community, but that once it was there, within-community factors, such as the degree of social contact, dominated the spread of the disease. Further work supported this conclusion (Herring and Sattenspiel, 2003; Sattenspiel et al., 2000). Although their study focused on very small populations in a localized region, it is likely that the lack of fit of global models to the magnitude and duration of epidemics within communities is due to similar causes, i.e., that magnitude of epidemic peaks and durations of epidemics at the global scale are dominated by within region factors rather than the travel between regions.

One of the main questions to ask of the population-based models for geographic spread is whether they provide insights into how diseases spread across the landscape that go beyond those available from more traditional statistical analyses of prevalence patterns. This question is especially important in light of the difficulties in gaining access to adequate transportation data, in the difficulties of dealing with the many modes of transportation people use to travel from place to place, and in the difficulty in simplifying the necessarily complex data sets to a form that can actually be used by the models. As the preceding discussion suggests, it is not clear that the existing models have led to significant advances in our ability to *predict* patterns of geographic spread. Nonetheless, the models add to our understanding of how diseases spread across different geographic scales and, in combination with other techniques, may well improve our abilities to predict and control global and regional epidemics. In addition, now that these kinds of models are becoming tied more directly to estimates of the actual structure of global transportation networks, the next major world-wide epidemic should give us a clear indication of how much the improved data underlying the models have improved model predictions. Unfortunately, however, it is difficult to assess their value until they are tested by a real epidemic.

Population-based geographic models also have significant advantages over other types of models. Data on transportation, disease cases, population, and other variables of interest are usually collected by government authorities, and, even if they are collected from individuals, they are commonly aggregated into groups at some specified spatial scale (e.g., neighborhood, health district, city, state) before they are made available to researchers. Thus, models that are developed using populations defined at these same levels of aggregation need make fewer assumptions about unknown structures than individual-based models or models based on different levels of spatial aggregation. In addition, population-based models usually have explicit mathematical structures that are amenable to theoretical analyses that can provide additional insights into factors influencing epidemic spread. They are also generally easier to use and quicker to implement, so in the face of a major epidemic they can be developed and provide early predictions to use in initial responses until such time as more accurate predictions are available.

3.3 INDIVIDUAL-BASED INFLUENZA MODELS

As the name implies, individual-based models explicitly model the behavior of individuals within a population. As was discussed in the previous chapter, most such models are fully stochastic models that take into account the randomness of individual behaviors. The structure of these models is often inspired by the structure of population-based models that have been used to address similar questions, but the underlying mathematical structure of individual-based models is often not explicit and may not be able to be represented in any simple form. In general, individual-based models are usually highly computer-intensive and the rise in their use has occurred alongside the development of technological improvements in computer and software design.

3.3.1 Model structures and general results

Individual-based models have become much more common in recent years, but the earliest use of such models for the spread of influenza dates back to a series of publications by researchers at the University of Minnesota in the early 1970s (Ackerman et al., 1984; Elveback et al., 1971, 1976; Ewy et al., 1972). This work centered around a Monte Carlo stochastic simulation model that was developed to help design an immunization strategy for influenza. The model was based on a population of 1000 individuals, including preschool children, grade school children, high school students, young adults, and older individuals. Depending on age, each person belonged to three or four different mixing groups relevant for disease transmission, including families, play groups, clusters of families (corresponding to neighborhoods or small social groups), and schools. Mixing groups for adults (e.g., workplaces) were built into the model, but most simulations focused on transmission occurring among children and so adult mixing groups were not explicitly considered (Elveback et al., 1976). In an attempt to incorporate as much information on the biology of the virus as possible, the length of the latent and infectious periods, the occurrence of illness, and the response to vaccination were all assumed to be random variables. Furthermore, because of the importance of schools for transmission of the virus, the basic time unit was set at one day so that schools could be open for 5 days and closed for 2 as they are in actuality.

Simulations of this model were used to study the conditions influencing the spread of both the 1957-58 Asian flu epidemic and the 1968-69 Hong Kong flu epidemic, which were observed to affect communities very differently. In newly invaded communities, Asian flu epidemics began explosively among the school-age population but then declined, leaving 20-30% of school children still susceptible. Rates of illness in contacts within 10 days of the onset of illness in an index case (i.e., secondary attack rates) also suggested that within-family spread was limited. Hong Kong flu epidemics, however, did not break out explosively and age-specific attack rates in the community were fairly uniform. It appeared from both the simulation results and analysis of actual epidemics that schools were the primary focus of epidemic spread for the Asian flu, but of somewhat less importance during the Hong Kong flu epidemic (Ackerman et al., 1984; Dunn et al., 1959).

The main purpose of this study was to design a model that approximated fairly realistically the actual contact structures present within communities to evaluate the relative effectiveness of different immunization strategies. In particular, the model was used to look at whether mass immunization of school children in addition to immunization of older adults and high-risk groups would be an effective strategy to control outbreaks and, if so, whether attention should be focused primarily on elementary school children or on both elementary aged and preschool children. Results suggested that because of the strong school link for Asian flu epidemics, the best strategy in that case would be to focus all vaccinations of children on those of elementary school age, while for Hong Kong flu epidemics, once a certain proportion of elementary school aged children were vaccinated, the remainder of vaccinations could be given to children of any age with about the same impact.

It should be noted that although this model incorporated highly structured contact groups within the community, the questions for which it was designed addressed only within-community spread. In order to consider the geographic spread among communities the model would need to link several communities together, each with a similar basic structure, and that requires much more computer power than was available at the time of the original studies. Recently, however, several new studies have been published that describe individual-based models for the geographic spread of influenza. Stimulated by fears of a new world-wide pandemic of influenza, Ferguson et al. (2005) and Longini et al. (2005) used individual-based models within a geographic framework to evaluate possible containment strategies in the face of a newly evolved avian influenza strain in Thailand. These same groups have also used individual-based models to study the impact of intervention strategies implemented after failure of initial containment efforts in the United States (Ferguson et al., 2006; Germann et al., 2006) and in Great Britain (Ferguson et al., 2006).

We describe here the two Thailand studies to illustrate how the approach is being used. Longini et al. (2005) constructed a model population of 500,000 people allocated among 36 geographic regions distributed in a region about the size and density of modern rural Thailand. Each locality consisted of about 28 villages composed of around 138 households and including a total of about 500 people. As in a real landscape, villages tended to be clustered rather than distributed randomly in space, and households were clustered within the villages. Household sizes and the age distribution within the population as a whole and within households were chosen to match distributions derived from census data collected in modern rural Thailand in 2000. Mixing groups included adult work groups, play groups and preschool groups, elementary schools, and lower and upper secondary schools. Longini et al. assumed that workers only came into contact with a relatively small number of coworkers; hence, workplace mixing-group sizes were chosen to reflect the size of potential contact groups rather than actual workplace populations.

As described in Longini et al. (2005), distance functions based on observed patterns of school attendance and travel to work locations were used to distribute simulated individuals across space and assign them to particular schools and workplaces. Observed data indicated that the vast majority of movement within rural Thailand is highly localized. Consequently, around 80% of the population was assumed to travel less than 15 km to work, and nearly all the rest traveled between 16 and 30 km. In addition to work and school groups, the model also included larger social groups averaging 100 people, which were designed to reflect casual contact at temples, markets, shops, and other similar locations. One centrally located 40-bed community hospital was also included in the model, which allowed for the hospitalization of at least some people with symptomatic influenza. Each of the 36 localities also included one influenza case holding center of size 100 for use if and when the hospital was full. People were also allowed to go to the hospital for a reason unrelated to influenza.

Longini et al.'s model structure mimics many real-world structures (as does that in the Minnesota simulations described above) and illustrates how the local space in which individuals interact is a close intertwining of geographic proximity and social proximity. Models that are limited to just physical distance fail to capture a very important dimension in the human use of space.

Because the Longini et al. model focused on the spread of a newly evolved influenza strain, little information existed on actual estimates of disease-related parameters. Consequently, model parameter estimates were based on patterns observed during previous Asian and Hong Kong flu pandemics, with allowance given for the possibility of greater transmissibility and severity of a new strain. Sensitivity analyses were conducted to determine the impact of these parameters on disease patterns.

The overall purpose of the model was to attempt to predict the spread of the new strain and to evaluate the ability of specific interventions to prevent spread out of the source area. The specific interventions assessed included targeted antiviral prophylaxis (giving antiviral drugs to a predetermined group), quarantine, and pre-vaccination (vaccinating prior to the detection of an outbreak). Results showed that if transmissibility of the virus was low enough, targeted antiviral prophylaxis carried out either by treating the earliest symptomatic cases and their close contacts or by targeting a percentage of individuals within the geographic locale of symptomatic cases would effectively contain the epidemic. With higher rates of transmission, localized household quarantine would have to be implemented in conjunction with the use of antivirals. The use of vaccination prior to an outbreak of the disease improved the success of antiviral prophylaxis and household quarantine at even higher levels of transmission (Figure 3.5). Longini et al. (2005) also suggested that a stockpile of 100,000 to 1 million courses of antiviral drugs would be sufficient to reduce the spread of the epidemic within their model population of 500,000 individuals and limit its spread to the rest of the world.

This model clearly has a strong geographic component within its structure, but the questions of interest were centered more on limiting regional and global transmission rather than predicting the spread of the epidemic to particular localities. As the movies in the online supplementary material associated with Longini et al. (2005) show, with no intervention the epidemic spread quickly throughout the entire region with no clear patterns of geographic diffusion, but epidemic spread in the presence of interventions was largely limited to the locality with the initial case.

Ferguson et al. (2005) developed a spatially explicit model of the

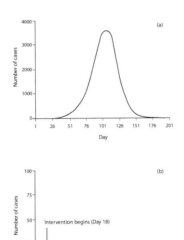

Figure 3.5 Smoothed curves approximating the results of simulations of the Longini et al. (2005) model with a) no interventions, and b) early interventions. Both sets of simulations assume that $R_0 = 1.4$.

spread of an avian influenza pandemic within the entire Thai population of 85 million and included also a 100-km-wide zone in countries bordering Thailand. Rather than incorporating distinct geographic localities, the Ferguson group used a map of the population density throughout their study region with a continuous, although spatially varying distribution of individuals. This map was derived from census, remote sensing, land use, and transportation data. Individuals within the simulated population were then assigned an age, household membership, and work or school membership. Similar to the model of Longini et al. (2005), the overall age distribution of the population, the size and distribution of households, the number, distribution, and assignments to workplaces or schools, and travel distances between home and work or school were allocated in accordance with known information about these characteristics within Thailand. Available disease data were used to derive new estimates of the incubation period for influenza and the pattern of infectivity, and other disease-related data were estimated using data from earlier influenza epidemics. Figure 3.6 shows simulations of an uncontrolled epidemic in Thailand using these parameter values and model structure.

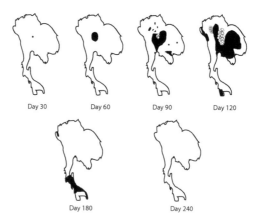

Figure 3.6 Example of a simulation showing the distribution of cases during an
uncontrolled influenza epidemic in Thailand using the Ferguson et al.
(2005) model with an R_0 of 1.5. Black areas represent hot spots of
infection, white circles represent recovered cases. The last two figures
omit recovered cases because they are distributed widely throughout
the country. See Ferguson et al. (2005) for the more detailed original
maps.

The primary goal of Ferguson et al. (2005) was essentially the same
as that of Longini and colleagues — to identify public health interventions that might be able to halt an epidemic shortly after its onset and
before it has a chance to spread to other regions. Ferguson et al. (2005)
also evaluated the effectiveness of targeted mass prophylactic use of
antiviral drugs, and they too looked at either giving the prophylaxis
to the social contacts of cases or targeting the entire population within
a certain geographic distance of cases. They did not include the use
of prevaccination, because they assumed that vaccines would not be
widely available in Thailand. Their analyses showed that geographic
targeting was more effective than purely social targeting, although
the effectiveness of either strategy or both combined was dependent
on how quickly clinical cases could be diagnosed and how efficiently
drugs could be distributed. Simulation results also suggested that
a stockpile of 3 million courses of antiviral drugs for the 85 million
people in Thailand in combination with measures such as quarantine
would be needed in order to achieve control of the epidemic.

3.3.2 Data issues and a brief critique of individual-based geographic models

Data issues are at least as important a concern for individual-based geographic models as for population-based models. Some data that are needed for such models are routinely collected in today's society. For example, information on a population's age distribution, the number of schools, the size of schools, and similar demographic data are easily accessible for the vast majority of the world's populations. Some types of data are not generally available except in rare circumstances. Thailand was chosen as the population to model in the two influenza studies discussed above not only because of its proximity to the source of a potentially deadly new strain of influenza, but also because an unusually large amount of information is known about the nature of social interactions on a daily basis within the country. Much of the stimulus for studies designed to collect such information was the AIDS epidemic and the clear recognition of the importance of social contact for the spread of that disease (see, for example, Morris et al., 1996; Wawer et al., 1996). However, although such data are a crucial component needed to guarantee that a complex individual-based model represents reality adequately, access to such data can be extremely difficult to arrange.

Data issues aside, one of the biggest problems associated with the use of individual-based geographic models is that in order to effectively address problems of interest, they are, of necessity, highly complex and computer intensive. They are expressly designed to reflect more closely the complexity and variability in behavior of actual groups of people than population-based models. They are difficult to design properly, both in terms of model structure and with regards to efficiency in computer programming, they are time-consuming and expensive to run unless the populations being modeled are extremely small (which severely limits their applicability to modern populations), and because they are generally fully stochastic in nature, simulations using a given parameter set must usually be run several hundreds to several thousands of times so that underlying patterns in the data will be revealed. The models are also difficult for others to reproduce and so their results cannot be verified easily.

In spite of all these concerns, individual-based models are an important step forward in the study of epidemic spread in human populations. Real human populations are composed of individuals who vary in their personal characteristics, their responses to what is going on around them, their biological reactions to invading microorganisms,

and their ability to pass those organisms on to others. It is essential
to explore the consequences of these known variations in order to better understand exactly what drives the spread of epidemics through
space. It is also important to attempt to take account of these factors
in trying to design appropriate strategies for containment and control
so that the world will be better able to deal with an epidemic, like
the 1918-19 influenza, that might have the potential to kill tens of
millions of people if left unchecked.

3.4   SO WHAT KIND OF MODEL SHOULD ONE USE TO STUDY INFLUENZA TRANSMISSION?

The studies described in this chapter illustrate clearly that our understanding of how influenza epidemics spread across time and space has
come from the results of both population-based and individual-based
models. As such, it can be difficult to decide which approach to take
when modeling the disease. Ultimately that decision must depend on
the specific questions the model is intended to address and on the
nature of the population being modeled. Population-based models
are almost always much easier to implement and, although they often require high-quality data sources that may be difficult to access,
the simplifying assumption that all individuals can be represented as
identical, ideal individuals reduces those needs significantly. Furthermore, if the intent is to gain good, theoretical understanding of the
impact of different factors on disease spread, then population-based
models may well be adequate for the purpose.

The majority of population-based models that are used in applications to human diseases are deterministic in structure, and so do not
incorporate enough of the stochasticity operating in real-world populations, however. The underlying methods used in these deterministic
models are based on assumptions that the modeled populations are
large enough that random effects can be ignored. If the intent of a
model is to explore a situation where stochastic factors are likely to be
of strong importance, then it is probably best to use at least a stochastic population-based model, if not an individual-based model. Good
theoretical insights may be possible using a deterministic population-
based model as a first approximation, but reasonable predictions and
full understanding of the factors influencing disease transmission call
for the use of models that incorporate the stochastic elements that
pervade real situations.

The population-based and individual-based models described in this chapter all looked at the geographic spread of influenza, but they are not fully comparable. Primarily this is because the questions being addressed by the models are fundamentally different, not only because the studies focused on different questions, but also because the questions themselves helped to select the appropriate methods. Most population-based influenza models have been concerned with explorations of how regional or global transportation helps to create broad observed patterns of epidemic spread. It is a daunting task to develop a truly individual-based model that encompasses all the individual variation at a world-wide scale, so collapsing the world or a large region into a manageable number of discrete cities or smaller regions is a reasonable strategy to take. On the other hand, effective containment strategies are nearly impossible to implement once an epidemic has spread world-wide and must almost certainly be focused on localized hot spots. Individual-based models, with their inherent random and localized structure may be better able to point out both the probable identification of hot spots and the best approaches to take to guarantee that enough individual chains of disease transmission can be stopped so that an epidemic will die out.

Chapter Four

Modeling Geographic Spread I:

Population-based Approaches

As the discussion of influenza models in the previous chapter showed, the distribution of populations across space and the patterns of interaction that link groups are important influences on how infectious diseases spread across time and space. In this chapter we describe in more detail the types of population-based models that have been developed to examine these influences. The main focus of our discussion will be on elucidating the general structures that have been used and the questions these models have addressed. In general, we will not include details on the analysis of these models; rather, we will largely limit our discussion to the kinds of results derived from the analyses and their importance in addressing questions related to the geographic spread of infectious diseases. Our primary intent is to introduce the large body of literature in this area in a way that will be accessible to readers with varied backgrounds and to stimulate at least some to delve deeper into the study of this important and interesting topic.

4.1 SPATIAL STRUCTURE AND DISEASE TRANSMISSION: BASIC THEMES

Epidemiologists have long been interested in the geographic distribution and spread of infectious diseases. One of the earliest formal studies of this was the influential work of John Snow in trying to understand the reasons underlying the distribution of cholera cases during an 1854 epidemic in London. As part of his work he mapped the spatial distribution of cholera cases, and noted the high degree of spatial localization of cases (see Figure 4.1). Upon further investigation of the patterns of water use of families with affected individuals he was able to trace the cholera to a particular water source. This pattern of localized transmission is a characteristic element of the majority of infectious disease epidemics that are spread through person to person contact or by means of a particular localized environmental feature.

In marked contrast to situations where populations might be well-mixed (a common assumption of models without spatial structure), local disease spread means that most of the population is not exposed to the infection immediately upon its introduction. Rather, the disease may have to pass through many intermediate individuals before reaching all members of the population. In addition, locally structured populations often exhibit clique behavior. For example, two people who are friends often have other friends in common, which reduces the opportunity for secondary infection events (Keeling et al., 1997). At a larger scale, residents of communities that are close together in space are likely to come into contact with each other more frequently than residents of communities that are more distant. As well as reducing the speed at which a disease spreads, local transmission leads to spatial clustering of disease cases such as that observed by John Snow, particularly during the early stages of an epidemic. Thus, introducing spatial structure into an epidemic model is essential whenever the questions of interest focus on initial epidemic spread, the impact of local interactions and environments, or similar factors.

Spatial structure also has important implications for disease persistence. In Chapter 2, we discussed how stochastic effects, such as demographic stochasticity, often lead to disease extinction, particularly in the period following a major epidemic when the number of individuals in a population who are susceptible to infection may be very small. As we discuss further in Section 4.3.2.3 and in later chapters, spatial heterogeneity can offset these effects — even if the infection undergoes fadeout in some locales, linkages between different locales can lead to repeated reintroductions, preventing permanent extinctions of the disease (Bolker and Grenfell, 1995, 1996) and enhancing the persistence of a disease at a regional level.

These "rescue" effects are most likely to occur if epidemics in different locations do not occur simultaneously, i.e., if there is some degree of asynchrony between locations. Much attention has been directed towards describing and understanding the degree to which epidemics occur synchronously in different locales (Bolker and Grenfell, 1996; Cliff et al., 1992a,b; Earn et al., 2000a,b; Earn and Levin, 2006; Grenfell et al., 2001; Keeling and Rohani, 2002; Lloyd and May, 1996; Lloyd and Jansen, 2004; Rohani et al., 1999) and to assessing the role asynchrony plays in generating observed patterns, especially in comparison with other potential factors such as the age distribution of populations or seasonally varying transmission rates. These

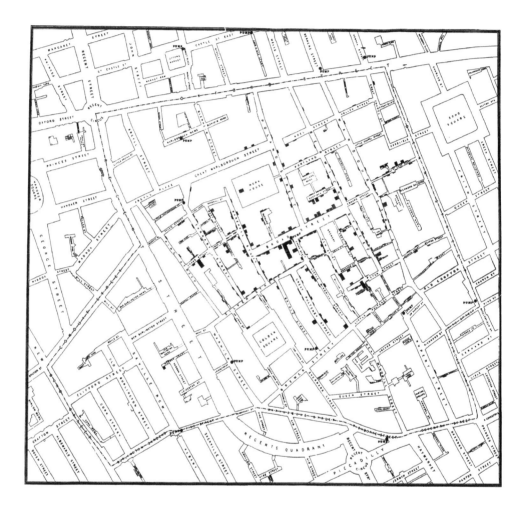

Figure 4.1 John Snow's map of the distribution of cholera cases in the Soho area of London during the 1854 epidemic. Cholera cases are represented by solid bars.

questions have been addressed extensively in studies of the cycling of measles over time and space, particularly in the United Kingdom and the United States; this interesting body of research is the focus of Chapter 5.

Besides influencing rates of spread and persistence of infections, the spatial nature of disease transmission has important consequences for control measures aimed at a disease. As the discussions in our applications chapters illustrate, a variety of control measures have been brought into play to help stem the course of major epidemics, including, for example, vaccination strategies, use of prophylactic drugs, culling of livestock, or quarantine. From an epidemiological point of view, if disease spread is mainly local in nature, control policies that target the local region in which the disease is concentrated and the surrounding area are likely to be more effective than measures that are imposed uniformly across the entire population (May and Anderson, 1984). It is important to remember, however, that epidemiological concerns, although of primary importance, are not the only issues that rise to the surface when humans are faced with uncontrolled epidemics. In 2001 the U.K. experienced a major epidemic of foot-and-mouth disease that nearly destroyed the nation's cattle industry. Epidemic modelers were asked to contribute to the task of determining strategies to use in combating the disease. The implications of local transmission for the effectiveness of suggested control policies played a central part in these efforts (Ferguson et al., 2001a; Keeling et al., 2001). However, much serious discussion ensued about the drastic nature of the response by authorities and whether such a response was truly needed. Chapter 7 is devoted to a discussion of this epidemic, the models that were developed to help veterinary public health efforts, the role models actually played in the effort to control the epidemic, and the aftermath of the epidemic, when all of the responses, including strategies based on both model results and traditional public health practices, were critically assessed. For now, though, we focus on the general types of population-based models that researchers have used in the pursuit of understanding how epidemics spread across space.

4.2 SPATIAL MODELING FRAMEWORKS

In many respects, spatial structure can be seen as just one type of heterogeneity to be included within a model — it serves to divide up a larger population into smaller components. Other sources of heterogeneity include, for example, age of individuals within populations or the types of risk behaviors individuals engage in. The standard modeling frameworks can easily be extended, in ways similar to those previously discussed, to include a description of the spatial structure of a population. Various modifications are possible, depending on the spatial scale of interest and the level of detail at which the population is to be modeled.

Our discussion of the characteristics of spatial models will extend over two chapters. In this chapter we describe the major population-based approaches; in chapter 6 we extend our discussion to individual-based approaches. The majority of population-based approaches fall under one of two types: 1) metapopulation or patch models, and 2) spatially continuous models. The Baroyan-Rvachev flu model and its variants described in the previous chapter are examples of the former type of model; models that consider patterns of diffusion of epidemics across landscapes often use formulations that are spatially continuous. Individual-based spatial models generally fall under the broad type called network models.

It is important to note that it is difficult to classify models into distinct classes: the divisions between different types of models are not clear-cut. For example, spatially continuous models are often discretized for simulation purposes, with space being subdivided into a number of cells. Such models could be viewed as metapopulation models. Metapopulation models can be viewed as network models in which the basic unit of description is a community or small population of individuals. Indeed, as the number of groups (or patches) in a metapopulation model increases, the model approaches an individual-based network model. Nonetheless, our categorization, although imperfect, should help in thinking about and understanding the differences and similarities among the various spatial modeling approaches.

4.3 METAPOPULATION MODELS

A metapopulation model is a particular type of multigroup model in which a population is distributed into a collection of n spatially discrete groups that are linked to one another in some way. Most often it is assumed that the individuals within a group are well mixed and that the groups or subpopulations are coupled to one another in some way. Coupling terms are used to represent the way that infection can be spread between groups. The spatial scale represented by the groups depends on the context of the study. For example, Baroyan et al. (1969) considered the groups to be different cities in Russia, while Sattenspiel and Hérring (1998) let each group represent small fur trapping communities in central Canada.

The number of variables needed to describe the state of a spatial metapopulation system is n times as many as is needed to describe a single well-mixed group, representing a considerable increase in the dimensionality of the model. As the number of groups in a metapopulation model is increased, it will at some point become comparable to the number of individuals in the population. In that case, the model might just as well be described in terms of the individual.

The metapopulation formulation is particularly well suited as a description of hierarchically structured populations (Cliff and Haggett, 1988; Cliff et al., 1993; Ferguson et al., 1997; Grenfell and Bolker, 1998; Grenfell et al., 2001; Haggett, 1982; May and Anderson, 1984; Murray and Cliff, 1977; Sattenspiel, 1987a,b; Sattenspiel and Simon, 1988; Watts et al., 2005). For instance, one might model a region consisting of one large population center, smaller satellite towns, and outlying rural areas, with coupling terms that represent the potential for spread between the city and the smaller satellite towns, and between the towns and rural areas. Such models are a reasonable description of many settings and have been widely employed, particularly in the geographic literature (see Chapter 8 for a more detailed discussion of geographic approaches). Many studies have focused on how hierarchical transmission impacts disease dynamics. For example, Sattenspiel (1987a,b) assigned individuals to a particular neighborhood and in addition, most individuals were also assigned to a day care facility in which they could interact with individuals from the same or other neighborhoods. Sattenspiel and Simon (1988) presented an analysis of the threshold behavior of this model. To capture the same sort of hierarchical behavior, Watts et al. (2005) recently developed a model that explicitly allows individuals to interact at multiple scales — all members are assigned to a particular local population, but in addition they can travel to a number of other contexts (schools, hospitals, other cities, etc.). Watts et al. then looked specifically at how such structure affects the basic reproductive number, R_0. A number of studies have addressed the potential for a large population center to drive epidemics in smaller centers that are connected to it (Cliff and Haggett, 1988; Grenfell and Bolker, 1998; Grenfell et al., 2001; Schwartz, 1992). Another interesting situation arises when fadeouts are frequent in the small towns, but the disease is maintained in the large city: the disease then undergoes frequent extinction in the towns followed by reintroduction (see, for example Cliff and Haggett, 1988;

Grenfell et al., 2001).

4.3.1 Formulation of metapopulation models

Metapopulation models can be separated into two approaches, which we designate as the mobility metapopulation approach and the cross-coupled metapopulation approach. The majority of metapopulation models used in studying the geographic spread of human infectious diseases are cross-coupled models. These models do not incorporate explicit mobility among groups; rather, they attempt to mimic the effect of explicit mobility by defining an appropriate contact matrix that represents the strength of contact within and between groups. The use of this approach dates to at least the mid-1940s; notable early examples include Murray and Cliff (1977); Rushton and Mautner (1955) and Wilson and Worcester (1945b).

The contact matrix at the heart of cross-coupled models, sometimes referred to as the WAIFW ("who acquires infection from whom") matrix, has elements that combine the effects of both contact and transmission within and between groups. Notice that as many as n^2 parameters are required to completely describe the mixing pattern. Consequently, simplified mixing patterns are often employed in applications and analyses of such models. In many cases, the WAIFW matrix is taken to be symmetric, and it is usually assumed that between-group transmission is less frequent than within-group transmission. Another common assumption is that contact between groups is a function of the distance between and/or size of the groups. Many studies simplify even further and reduce the WAIFW matrix to a form that depends on as few as two parameters (the between- and within-group transmission parameters). For instance, it might be assumed that the between-group coupling is identical between any distinct pair of groups, or that coupling only occurs between neighboring groups. Examples of additional simplified WAIFW matrices are described below in Section 4.3.2.1.

A deterministic SIR cross-coupled metapopulation model can be written as the following set of differential equations:

$$\dot{S}_i = \mu N_i - \mu S_i + S_i \sum_{j=1}^{n} \frac{\phi_{ij} I_j}{N_i} \tag{4.1}$$

$$\dot{I}_i = S_i \sum_{j=1}^{n} \frac{\phi_{ij} I_j}{N_i} - (\mu + \gamma) I_i . \tag{4.2}$$

The ϕ_{ij} form the elements of the WAIFW matrix.

Mobility metapopulation models are mechanistically oriented and explicitly incorporate movement of individuals between groups (see, for example, Ball, 1991; Bartlett, 1956; Baroyan and Rvachev, 1967; Sattenspiel and Dietz, 1995). This movement can be either permanent migration or temporary mobility, with the latter often of more importance for directly transmitted human diseases. Transmission of infection occurs within groups, but those groups consist of a mixture of individuals, some of whom are residents of the group and some of whom are visitors.

In a general mobility metapopulation model, the basic description of mobility involves specifying the (per capita) rate at which individuals leave each group and the destinations of these individuals. Since there are n groups, this requires n^2 additional parameters compared to the nonspatial model. If the mobility is temporary rather than permanent, it is also necessary to specify return rates. As in the cross-coupled models, in many cases simplified descriptions of mobility are employed to reduce the number of parameters needed to specify the spatial structure. For instance, the rate at which individuals leave a group might be assumed to be the same for all groups, and a particularly simple pattern of mobility might be employed, such as movement to nearest neighbors or equally likely movement to any other group.

One example of a deterministic SIR mobility metapopulation model is the following set of differential equations:

$$\dot{S}_i = \mu N_i - \frac{\beta_i S_i I_i}{N_i} - \mu S_i + \sum_{j=1}^{n} \theta_{ij}^{(S)} S_j \qquad (4.3)$$

$$\dot{I}_i = \frac{\beta_i S_i I_i}{N_i} - (\mu + \gamma) I_i + \sum_{j=1}^{n} \theta_{ij}^{(I)} I_j . \qquad (4.4)$$

S_i and I_i denote the numbers of susceptible and infectious individuals in the different groups, respectively. The transmission parameter for each group is written as β_i and the population size of a group is given by N_i. Movement between groups is described by the dispersal parameters $\theta_{ij}^{(X)}$. Notice that the dispersal parameters can be allowed to be dependent on an individual's disease status. Notice also that disease transmission (represented by β) and mobility (represented by the dispersal parameters) are separate terms in this model. Baroyan and Rvachev (1967), Bartlett (1956), and Sattenspiel and Dietz (1995) assumed that individuals in any disease state were able to move among groups, but mathematical analysis of this kind of model is difficult. In an effort to simplify the analysis, Ball (1991) assumed that only infectious individuals were allowed to move between groups.

In mobility models, movement of individuals between groups can take many different forms, including transient visits of varying lengths, after which individuals return to their home group (examples of this might include a day's visit to a neighboring town or village) or permanent moves from one group to another (e.g., moving a household from one town to another). Some descriptions, therefore, divide the population of a given group into residents and visitors (Keeling and Rohani, 2002; Sattenspiel and Dietz, 1995). If individuals return home following a visit, visitors must be labeled according to their home group (Sattenspiel and Dietz, 1995). Note that in such a formulation the inclusion of spatial structure results in n^2 as many state variables (or population classes) as in the corresponding nonspatial model.

An important, but obvious, point to notice is that in mobility models individuals are only present in a single group at a time: they cannot be involved in the epidemic process in two different groups simultaneously. This is not always true for the cross-coupled model — with many definitions of the contact matrix, coupling between groups leads to an increase in the number of contacts made by an individual. (This essentially corresponds to individuals spending part of their time in two or more groups at once.) Thus, in some formulations of the cross-coupled model, the basic reproductive number, R_0, increases with the strength of coupling between groups. It is always possible to rescale the transmission parameter appropriately to counteract this behavior, however.

Although the cross-coupling and mobility formulations appear to be quite different, there are similarities between them. Ball (1991) demonstrated an equivalence between the two formulations — albeit for the case in which only infectious individuals migrate between groups — and he also provided an explicit way to convert the parameter set from one of his formulations into an appropriate set for the other. This reparameterization is determined by equating the forces of infection felt in each group within the two formulations. Ball further showed that the final sizes of epidemics in both formulations were the same, although the time courses of the epidemics could differ.

Ball (1991) illustrated the different time courses that could result from the two models by using his methodology to examine the speed of epidemic waves resulting from the two frameworks. If the groups are arranged linearly, Ball's reparameterization method can be used to produce a pair of metapopulation models that mimic spatially discrete versions of either a cross-coupled metapopulation model or a mobility metapopulation model with nearest-neighbor coupling. The cross-coupled metapopulation model exhibits faster waves than the equivalent mobility metapopulation model, since the former allows for some long-range contacts. Working along the same lines, Keeling and Rohani (2002) showed that, in the vicinity of an equilibrium solution, the eigenvalues describing the linearizations of these two models could be mapped onto each other by an appropriate choice of parameters. This mapping can be performed explicitly using the results of Lloyd and Jansen (2004), which provide analytic expressions for the eigenvalues.

4.3.2 Common questions addressed using metapopulation models

Metapopulation models have been used extensively in studies of infectious disease transmission and control within a spatial framework. Much of this work considers the impact of infectious diseases in wild and domesticated plant and animal populations and is largely outside the scope of this book. Because application of these models to the study of human infectious diseases is covered in some detail in Chapters 3, 5, and 7, in this section we focus on introducing several of the common questions related to the spread of human infectious diseases that are examined using metapopulation models.

4.3.2.1 Coupling patterns in metapopulation models

Both cross-coupled metapopulation models and mobility metapopulation models have at their core a structure that serves to link the different subpopulations to one another. This kind of structure is often called the coupling pattern because it indicates the strength of the interaction (or coupling) between each pair of subpopulations. Recall that the major distinction between the two is that mobility models explicitly incorporate movement of individuals between groups while cross-coupled models do not. In cross-coupled models the strength of interactions between groups is designated by the modeler (in the form of the WAIFW matrix), while in mobility models the rates of travel or mixing between different of groups are designated and the strength of the interaction between two specific groups is an outcome of the mixing process within the entire population.

Measurement of the coupling between groups in either kind of metapopulation model is often difficult, primarily because it involves detailed data on interactions between groups and these data are often not available. Consequently, modelers frequently make simplifying assumptions about the nature of between-group coupling and about the groups themselves. To illustrate the kinds of assumptions commonly made, we limit our discussion to cross-coupled models since it is much easier to describe the structure of the WAIFW matrix than it is to describe the group interactions resulting from a mobility process.

As mentioned above, the most common of these assumptions are that each group is of equal size $(N_i = N)$, that the degree of interaction between-groups is smaller than the degree of interaction within groups, and that the coupling matrix is symmetric. Two types of symmetric coupling matrices are frequently used in the literature. In the first case it is assumed that the between-group coupling is equal for all pairs of groups. This generates the following coupling matrix (which we call "equal between-group coupling" to facilitate comparison with other patterns):

$$\begin{pmatrix} 1 & \epsilon & \epsilon & \epsilon \\ \epsilon & 1 & \epsilon & \epsilon \\ \epsilon & \epsilon & 1 & \epsilon \\ \epsilon & \epsilon & \epsilon & 1 \end{pmatrix}$$

ϵ can be thought of as a scaling factor that tells how much between-group contact is changed relative to within-group contact. As a consequence of the assumption that between-group interactions are less common than within-group interactions, the value of ϵ must be a number between zero and one, and it is usually assumed further that it is small. The rates of transmission within and between groups are then found by multiplying the appropriate element of the coupling matrix by β, the within-group transmission parameter. Note that in this model the within-group transmission parameters are given by $\beta \cdot 1 = \beta$, which is equal to the transmission parameter of the non-spatial model, while the between-group transmission parameters are equal to $\beta \cdot \epsilon$.

A second common model for the coupling matrix is that of nearest-neighbor coupling. In this model each group interacts only with its neighbors. The simplest models of this type assume that the groups are arranged in a linear fashion, but this means that the groups at the ends of the line would only have one neighbor each. Consequently, sometimes it is assumed that the groups are arranged in a circle so that all groups have two neighbors. Assume again that the between-group coupling occurs at a rate ϵ. Then the linear version of the nearest-neighbor coupling matrix would have the following form:

$$\begin{pmatrix} 1 & \epsilon & 0 & 0 \\ \epsilon & 1 & \epsilon & 0 \\ 0 & \epsilon & 1 & \epsilon \\ 0 & 0 & \epsilon & 1 \end{pmatrix}$$

while the circular version of the matrix would be

$$\begin{pmatrix} 1 & \epsilon & 0 & \epsilon \\ \epsilon & 1 & \epsilon & 0 \\ 0 & \epsilon & 1 & \epsilon \\ \epsilon & 0 & \epsilon & 1 \end{pmatrix}$$

As in the example of equal coupling between groups, the rates of transmission within and between groups are found by multiplying the appropriate element of the coupling matrix by β.

Many other coupling matrices have been used in studying various diseases. The mixing patterns described in Chapter 2 are examples of additional ways to think about coupling between subpopulations.

4.3.2.2 The basic reproductive number for metapopulation models

As is the case in most epidemic models, the first step in the analysis of many metapopulation models is the determination of R_0, the basic reproductive number. This task is much more difficult for metapopulation and other structured population models than for homogeneous single-population models. Early attempts relied on simplifications of the model structures. For example, Hethcote and Van Ark (1987), Lloyd and May (1996), and May and Anderson (1984) were able to estimate R_0 for simple cross-coupled systems with equally sized groups and a WAIFW matrix of simple form. A major advance in this area was made by Diekmann et al. (1990), who derived a general procedure for calculating the R_0 associated with epidemic models; their approach is outlined in Section 2.5. Drawing on this method, van den Driessche and Watmough (2002) focused in on models that specifically incorporated heterogeneous subgroups and presented a precise definition of R_0 that could be used for models incorporating a variety of heterogeneous structures (e.g., age groups or populations separated in space). The methods of Diekmann et al. (1990) and van den Driessche and Watmough (2002) are now being used on a regular basis to determine R_0 for metapopulation models. This process is fairly straightforward for cross-coupled models, but a little more complex for mobility metapopulation models because in mobility models infectious individuals can move back and forth between different groups over the course of their infectious period (see Arino and van den Driessche (2003), Arino et al. (2005), or Fulford et al. (2002) for examples of the latter). Readers interested in the details of how to calculate R_0 for both structured and unstructured models are encouraged to consult Diekmann et al. (1990) and van den Driessche and Watmough (2002).

4.3.2.3 Cycling, persistence, synchrony, and metapopulation models

Disease fadeout is a significant feature of the epidemiology of many infectious diseases, and it is especially important in understanding long-term temporal trends of many human diseases (present and past), such as measles, pertussis, or smallpox. The time series of such diseases is characterized by distinct cycling in the incidence of the disease, with the period of the cycles being a characteristic associated with each disease. For example, Jorde et al. (1990) showed that smallpox epidemics in Finland occurred about every 5 years between 1751 and 1824, but the interepidemic period extended to 7.4 years between 1825 and 1920, primarily because of the introduction of widespread vaccination for the disease. As is common in many similar diseases, between epidemics the disease prevalence was reduced to very low levels and in many cases the disease died out.

One issue related to the long-term cycling of epidemics in a geographic context is the question of whether outbreaks in the different patches or communities making up the larger population are synchronized with one another. Intuitively, it is easy to see that if a disease dies out at about the same time in all groups, then it will die out in the population as a whole. If the timing of die out varies among groups, however, then contact with groups that are actively experiencing an outbreak can reintroduce the disease into groups in which it has died out. Thus, asynchrony in outbreaks over a geographic region can enhance persistence of the disease within that region.

Observation of the incidence of many human diseases indicates that they do not appear to die out over time (see Figure 5.2, for example; many other diseases show similar patterns). This observation has motivated a large number of studies aimed at identifying and assessing the importance of underlying causes of synchrony and asynchrony in disease outbreaks (see, for example, Bolker and Grenfell, 1996; Cliff et al., 1992a,b; Earn et al., 2000a,b; Earn and Levin, 2006; Grenfell et al., 2001; Keeling and Rohani, 2002; Lloyd and May, 1996; Lloyd and Jansen, 2004; Rohani et al., 1999). Metapopulation models have been used extensively to address these issues and they have significantly advanced our understanding of the reasons for disease fadeout, synchrony of epidemics, and epidemic cycling. Metapopulation models have also been used to help assess the degree to which outbreaks in certain locales lag behind or lead ahead of those in other locales and to understand the underlying reasons for such behavior (Cliff et al., 1992a,b; Grenfell et al., 2001). We provide extensive discussion of how these models have advanced our understanding of measles epidemiology in the next chapter; here we present an introduction to the basic mathematical concepts underlying those applications.

One factor that can have a strong influence on whether disease outbreaks become synchronized within a region is seasonality in disease transmission rates and other parameters. If seasonal effects are significant for a particular disease, they will tend to lead to increased synchronization among groups residing in similar environments since those groups would experience increased risks for disease at similar times. At smaller geographic scales, groups are more likely to reside in similar environments, and so in such situations the synchronizing effects of seasonal variations in parameter values will be greater.

The level of coupling between communities also affects the chance that outbreaks will become synchronized. This relationship has been studied by a number of researchers. For example, using a technique previously developed for ecological models, Jansen and Lloyd (2000) and Lloyd and Jansen (2004) separated model behavior into a collection of modes, one of which corresponded to in-phase behavior (where the numbers of infectious individuals in each group oscillate together), with the others describing out-of-phase behavior (where the groups do not oscillate together). Their analysis showed that, provided the spatial coupling was not extremely weak, the out-of-phase modes decayed rapidly, leaving the in-phase mode as the dominant behavior of the system. Thus, their results indicated that synchrony should often be expected in metapopulation models. Lloyd and Jansen (2004) showed that these results were similar for both cross-coupled and mobility metapopulation models, as long as the mobility rates in the latter did not depend on the disease status of individuals.

The level of coupling also influences the probability of disease fadeout. For example, Keeling (2000a) used a methodological technique based on moment equations to predict the persistence of a disease at the regional level. He showed that if spatial coupling is too weak, recolonization is an infrequent event, causing the disease to die out at the regional level. If spatial coupling is too strong, however, groups become synchronized and so are likely to undergo extinction at the same time, reducing the opportunity for recolonization to occur. His results thus indicate that disease persistence is most likely when levels of spatial coupling are intermediate.

Finally, as discussed in Section 2.4.3, stochasticity plays an important role in disease fadeout, particularly early or late in an epidemic when the number of infectious individuals is very small. It is also particularly important in small populations. Small populations do not tend to experience the long-term cycling of diseases like smallpox and measles; rather, the basic pattern is one of severe epidemics interspersed with disease-free periods of variable length (Cliff et al., 1981). Often epidemics can be tied to specific events allowing reintroduction of the pathogen into the region (see, for example, Mielke et al. (1984)).

4.3.2.4 Hierarchical transmission through metapopulations: cities, towns, and villages

Metapopulation models are particularly well-suited to studying how the types of economic and social relationships among human communities affect patterns of disease spread. Some of the earliest work of this type is the Russian flu modeling of Baroyan, Rvachev, and colleagues described in the previous chapter, although this work focused more on the specific linkages derived from existing transportation data or assumptions about the transportation network than on the implications of general types of interactions among communities. Human activities are often structured in broadly similar ways in different regions, however, and these activities commonly result in a settlement pattern such that there are one or two major cities or towns of moderate to large size that serve as market centers or centers of activity for the entire region. Surrounding these major communities are a number of smaller towns and villages that are weakly to moderately coupled to the major center, but that interact only rarely with other small towns and villages.

The consequences for disease transmission of this kind of structure have received much attention within the metapopulation framework. May and Anderson (1984), building on work of Hethcote (1978) and Post et al. (1983), developed an epidemic model for this kind of situation, which they termed the "cities and villages" model. They used this model to study the impact of vaccination (or some other disease control measure) in such a setting. In particular, they addressed the question of whether it would be better to vaccinate individuals in the city or in the villages. Their model showed that a uniform vaccination policy, in which the same fraction of individuals is vaccinated in each population center — regardless of size — required that a larger fraction of the population be vaccinated than would be predicted by (incorrectly) assuming that the population was well mixed. Consequently, the optimal vaccination policy would be one that involved vaccinating a larger proportion of individuals in the city than in the smaller villages. May and Anderson (1984) concluded that by taking advantage of the heterogeneity within the region, disease eradication could be achieved with a lower population-level vaccination fraction than would be predicted under the perfect mixing assumption.

Hethcote and Van Ark (1987) pointed out problems related to the dependence of transmission parameters on the relative sizes of the cities and villages in May and Anderson's study, and so they suggested a need to modify the transmission terms. This modification reduces the differences between vaccination programs observed by May and Anderson (1984), but the qualitative conclusions still stand. Uniform vaccination policies perform worse than those that target larger population centers.

Sattenspiel et al. (2000) looked more generally at the impact of different idealized, but reasonable geographic structures resulting from the economic and social relationships linking different communities within a region. In particular, they used a mobility metapopulation model to study the impact of four different mobility schemes on the patterns of spread within a region. These models included the following: 1) a Frontier scenario, which might apply to communities in a frontier situation where residents of a large community leave to found successively smaller communities at greater distances from the largest community (Figure 4.2a), 2) a Central Marketplace scenario, similar to May and Anderson's "cities and villages" scenario, where outlying communities are linked to the central community but not to each other (Figure 4.2b), 3) a Sister Towns scenario where outlying communities are more likely to interact with other outlying communities than they are to interact with the largest community (Figure 4.2c), and 4) a Circuit scenario, where communities interact only with their nearest neighbors in a circular fashion (Figure 4.2d). Results from the analysis of these different idealized patterns suggested that communities with a central location in the social and political hierarchy of a region may play a more important role in influencing patterns of epidemic spread than communities that are centrally located geographically but not socially.

The dynamical impact of coupling a large population center to smaller outlying communities has also been of much interest, particularly in regard to the transmission dynamics of measles. As measles modeling is discussed at length in Chapter 5, we defer detailed discussion of the disease until then. The most important observation is that if the population of the city is large enough to make stochastic extinction unlikely, the population-level dynamics in the outlying regions are dominated by repeated local extinction, followed by reintroduction (Cliff and Haggett, 1988; Grenfell et al., 2001). This leads to waves of infection traveling outwards from the large population center into the rural hinterland.

4.4 SPATIALLY CONTINUOUS MODELS

We now turn to the second major type of population-level spatial model — spatially continuous models. These models assume that the population is continuously distributed across space rather than distributed into several discrete subpopulations. The spatial location is represented by the variable $\mathbf{x}$, and the densities of susceptible and infectious individuals at any time t throughout the region are represented by $S(\mathbf{x}, t)$ and $I(\mathbf{x}, t)$.

The spatially continuous framework is quite flexible, and so contains a spectrum of models of varying complexities. The earliest models were fairly basic, employing simple descriptions of the transmission process, but many refinements have since been described.

One advantage of the spatially continuous approach is that it is particularly amenable to mathematical analysis. These analyses, although largely theoretical in focus, have led to many important insights into the behavior of spatial models that have driven progress in understanding patterns of spatial spread of infectious disease, not only for spatially continuous scenarios, but also for other, more realistic scenarios. In the remainder of this chapter we introduce a few of the simplest spatially continuous models in order to illustrate the nature of this important class of epidemic models. We also discuss important properties that emerge from analyses of this class of models. Many of these properties relate to the nature of epidemic waves and their speed of spread along a landscape, and the basic ideas can be illustrated using the simplest spatially continuous models.

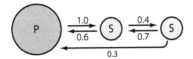

a) The Frontier scenario

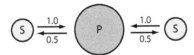

b) The Central Marketplace scenario

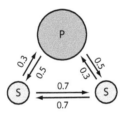

c) The Sister Towns scenario

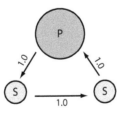

d) The Circuit scenario

Figure 4.2 Four idealized mobility schemes designed to reflect possible economic and social relationships linking neighboring communities. See text for descriptions of each scenario. Redrawn from Sattenspiel et al. (2000), Figure 3.

4.4.1 The reaction-diffusion model

In the most basic spatially continuous models, disease transmission is assumed to be a local event. This assumption means that the rate of transmission at a given point in space depends only on the densities of susceptible and infectious individuals at that point. If the disease process is assumed to follow the basic SIR model described in Chapter 2 with only the addition of the spatial dimension for densities of individuals, then the transmission process can be modeled as $\beta S(\mathbf{x}, t)I(\mathbf{x}, t)$ (note that because S and I are defined in terms of densities, it is not necessary to divide by the population size). If a modeler wants to allow the transmission risk to also vary spatially, then a simple assumption would be to allow the transmission parameter β to also be a function of space, i.e., $\beta(\mathbf{x}, t)$. Population mixing can then be introduced by allowing individuals to move about at random, as described, for instance, by a spatial random walk or diffusion process. Mathematically, such a process can be described deterministically by a diffusion equation. Together with the local description of infection, this gives rise to what is called a reaction-diffusion model for the spatial spread of a disease (Murray et al., 1986; Noble, 1974).

A simple deterministic SIR reaction-diffusion model without demography can be written as

$$\frac{\partial S(\mathbf{x}, t)}{\partial t} = -\beta S(\mathbf{x}, t)I(\mathbf{x}, t) + D_S \nabla^2 S(\mathbf{x}, t) \qquad (4.5)$$

$$\frac{\partial I(\mathbf{x}, t)}{\partial t} = \beta S(\mathbf{x}, t)I(\mathbf{x}, t) - \gamma I(\mathbf{x}, t) + D_I \nabla^2 I(\mathbf{x}, t). \qquad (4.6)$$

The first term of Equation 4.5 and the first two terms of Equation 4.6 describe the local processes of infection and recovery, while the last terms of each equation describe the diffusion of individuals across the landscape. The operator ∇^2 (called the Laplacian operator) gives the second derivative with respect to the spatial variables. For example, in one dimension the spatial position can be denoted by a single variable $\mathbf{x}$ and so $\nabla^2 = \partial^2/\partial x^2$. In two dimensions the spatial position is commonly denoted by the two variables $\mathbf{x}$ and $\mathbf{y}$ and so $\nabla^2 = \partial^2/\partial x^2 + \partial^2/\partial y^2$. The speed of the spatial diffusion is controlled by the two diffusion coefficients, D_S and D_I, which refer to the diffusion of the susceptible and infectious individuals, respectively. The simplest model would assume that these coefficients were equal for both groups; alterations of this assumption are commonly considered in the literature. Reaction-diffusion models have a long history in mathematical biology, most notably with the studies of Fisher (1937) and Kolmogoroff et al. (1937) on the spatial spread of an advantageous gene and the work of Turing (1952) on pattern formation via diffusion-driven instabilities.

Even within the reaction-diffusion setting, various versions of the model given by Equations 4.5 - 4.6 are considered in the literature.[1] For example, in their rabies model (discussed in more detail in Section 4.4.1.2), Murray et al. (1986) make the simplifying assumption that only infected animals disperse. In most reaction-diffusion epidemic models, it is assumed that the environment is homogeneous, so that the birth rate and the transmission parameter are constant across space. In addition, for many models the initial conditions are chosen in a simple way with, for instance, a spatially homogeneous susceptible population and initial infection restricted to some bounded area or even a single point. More complex models add in such characteristics as spatially varying demographic and/or transmission parameters, reflecting the possibility that certain areas of the environment may be more or less favorable for the host species or disease transmission. Complexity may also increase if the diffusion parameter is assumed to vary over space — an assumption that may be made to reflect natural boundaries in the environment (such as rivers or mountain ranges).

4.4.1.1 Invasion and traveling waves in reaction-diffusion models

One of the major questions asked of all epidemic models is whether a disease will be able to invade a population, and if that is the case, to whom it spreads (and where, in the case of spatial models) immediately following invasion of a population. In spatially continuous models, localized introduction of infection often leads to wave-like behavior as the disease spreads out from the initial focus. If you were to look at any given point in space (or in a small region), you would observe a typical epidemic time curve (assuming that there are no births to replenish the pool of susceptibles): following introduction of the disease, the epidemic takes off slowly, then increases rapidly to its peak, and then declines as the local population of susceptibles is depleted (Figure 4.3). Viewed over the entire region, the spread of the epidemic often occurs as a spatial wave, with most cases being found near the wave front but with very few cases far behind the front (because the epidemic has passed its peak in regions behind the front) (see, for example, Murray et al., 1986; Murray, 1989). In the simplest

---

[1]See Rass and Radcliffe (2003) for a recent survey of many of these models.

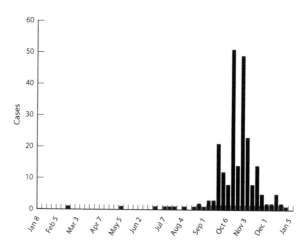

Figure 4.3 Epidemic curve showing reported measles cases during a 1984 measles epidemic in the Commonwealth of Dominica, West Indies.

models this wave front is circular in appearance.

Analysis of the model given by Equations 4.5 - 4.6 begins by looking for solutions that are traveling waves moving at speed c. The standard way to do this is to define a new variable $z = x - ct$, which shifts the coordinates of the system to a frame of reference that moves at speed c. From the perspective of the z coordinates, it looks as if you are sitting at the wave front and moving along with it in space and time rather than watching it pass you by (see Figure 4.4). As long as you are not too far behind the wave front, the model can be linearized by setting S equal to its initial density S_0. In this linearized model the number of infectious individuals I continues to grow exponentially as the wave front passes, because the depletion of susceptibles is ignored in the linearized model. Analysis of this model shows that there is a minimum wave speed, c_0, at which a traveling wave can move. This wave speed is given by the following:

$$c_0 = 2\sqrt{D_I(\beta S_0 - \gamma)} = 2\sqrt{D_I \gamma (R_0 - 1)}. \tag{4.7}$$

R_0 is the basic reproductive number and equals $\beta S_0 / \gamma$.

Murray (1989) shows that the epidemic wave actually travels at the minimum wave speed c_0. Thus, Equation 4.7 gives a simple relationship between the epidemiological parameters (R_0 and γ), the

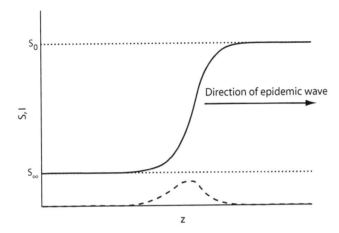

Figure 4.4 The spatial traveling wave seen in the reaction-diffusion SIR epidemic
model, assuming a spatially homogeneous environment. The solid curve
shows the density of susceptible individuals; the dashed curve shows the
density of infectious individuals.

diffusion coefficient for infectious individuals (D_I), and the resulting
wave speed (c).

It is important to remember that the linearized model cannot be a
good description of epidemic spread over arbitrarily long times. The
linear assumption means that under conditions of epidemic growth
(i.e., when $R_0 > 1$) the infective density will never stop growing behind the epidemic wave front. In reality, the behavior seen at any
point in space mirrors that described in Chapter 2 for simple nonspatial models. If there are no susceptible births, then the disease will die
out locally. If the pool of susceptibles is being replenished, however,
it may be possible to establish an endemic level of disease. As the
susceptible pool is replenished by births, epidemics can recur behind
the main front if infection remains. As discussed in Section 4.4.1.2,
however, the occurrence of such secondary epidemic waves may be
highly dependent on stochastic effects.

The full nonlinear model does not exhibit the unbounded growth
seen in the linearized model, since the depletion of susceptibles causes
the epidemic increase to slow and then decline. A natural question
to ask is what effect this has upon the wave behavior described for

the linearized model. The linear conjecture of van den Bosch et al. (1990) suggests that, under fairly general conditions, the nonlinear model exhibits wave-like solutions and the asymptotic wave speed is equal to the minimum wave speed, c_0, calculated using the appropriate linearization. This conjecture, which is supported by the observed behavior of a wide range of models, is said to be likely to hold if two assumptions are met. First, the interactions between individuals must be sufficiently localized and, secondly, the conditions in the infection-free population should be optimal for the infectious agent (Metz et al., 2000). Mollison (1991) remarks that the first assumption does not refer to long-distance dispersal of infectious individuals, but rather to certain nonlocal nonlinearities. He cites, as an example, a situation in which the infection probability is reduced across an entire region if the total number of infectious individuals reaches a threshold level. Such effects would not appear to be particularly relevant to most epidemic models, and so may only represent a technicality of the analysis.

The linearized and nonlinear deterministic models also differ somewhat in their correspondence with respective stochastic models. The behaviors of deterministic and stochastic versions of the linear model are related, in that the former gives the expected numbers of the corresponding stochastic process (Mollison, 1977, 1991). This observation, combined with the linear conjecture of van den Bosch et al. (1990), means that if calculation of the wave speed is the major question of interest, little extra information is gained by studying nonlinear deterministic or linear stochastic formulations of the model. Notice, however, that these formulations may provide additional information regarding certain features of the disease invasion process. For instance, the deterministic model does not address the question of whether stochastic effects might interrupt the epidemic process or provide estimates for how close individual epidemic realizations lie to the time course of their average.

The correspondence between the stochastic and deterministic models is more complex in the nonlinear case. Questions regarding the correspondence between nonlinear stochastic and deterministic models are typically addressed within the framework of individual-based formulations. A more detailed description of the behavior of such models appears in Chapter 6.

The linear model does provide an upper bound for the nonlinear epidemic (Mollison, 1991), because epidemic growth is slowed if the density of susceptibles is lower than the initial density assumed by the linear analysis. It is important to realize, however, that several different nonlinear models can share the same linearization. The linear theory will predict the same wave speed for each of these models, while in reality their wave speeds may well differ.

Mollison (1991) also points out that the dimensionality of space does not affect wave speed in the linear framework, whereas it often does in nonlinear models. An individual-based model for the simple epidemic process, in which individuals are situated on a lattice (square grid) with contact only between nearest neighbors and in which there is no recovery from the disease (i.e., individuals remain infectious forever once infected), provides an example. (See Chapter 6 for a more detailed discussion of such models.) For a particular set of parameters, the linearization predicts a wave speed of about 1.5 in either a one-dimensional (individuals situated on a line) or a two-dimensional (individuals situated on a regular square grid) setting. The wave speed in the corresponding nonlinear model does, however, differ between the one-dimensional (speed = 0.5) and two-dimensional (speed about 0.84) arrangements.

4.4.1.2 An example of the use of reaction-diffusion models — the Murray et al. (1986) rabies model

The spread of the rabies virus in wild animal populations has been an active area of epidemiologic research using reaction-diffusion models. In Europe, the main host for rabies is the red fox (*Vulpes vulpes*), although other mammals (including other fox species, dogs, and bats) are also important. In the U.S. and Canada, raccoons are a major host for the infection. Building on a nonspatial model (Anderson et al., 1981), which developed a basic description of the population dynamics of foxes and the transmission dynamics of rabies, Murray and colleagues developed a model for the spatial spread of rabies (Murray et al., 1986).

The major stimulus for the formation of the Anderson and Murray models was to assess the potential for spread after an introduction of rabies into Great Britain (the disease has been absent from the country since the early part of the 20th century). The reaction-diffusion model predicts wave-like spread, although spatial heterogeneity in the density of the fox population leads to a more complicated pattern of spread than is seen in the simplest models. For instance, as Figure 4.5 shows, following a point introduction, the wave front is not circular because the disease spreads more quickly in areas in which the density of foxes is high. This causes the wave front to take on a more scalloped appearance (Murray et al., 1986).

As discussed above, in the nonlinear model the local depletion of

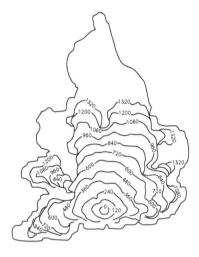

Figure 4.5 Wave of advance of rabies cases resulting from a simulation of the Murray et al. (1986) rabies model. Contour lines give the position of the wave front every 120 days. See original source for details on the model and parameter values used to generate the map. Redrawn from Murray et al. (1986), Figure 11.

susceptibles will cause local epidemics to wane, but if there is replenishment of the susceptible population through births, the susceptible population will eventually rise above the threshold. If infectious individuals are still present a second epidemic can be triggered, leading to a secondary traveling wave phenomenon. See Figure 12 in Murray et al. (1986) for an example of a simulation showing such a secondary wave.

As we saw in Chapter 2, in the nonspatial deterministic SIR model with demography it is possible for the number of infectious individuals to fall so low as to be a small fraction of an individual. When stochastic effects are taken into account, however, more realistic results follow in that extinction of the disease commonly occurs. This same kind of behavior applies to the spatial setting, and, in fact, it may be even more pronounced because spatial models consider the behavior of epidemics within local regions rather than in large, homogeneously mixing populations.

The Murray et al. (1986) rabies model can be criticized for similar reasons. For example, Mollison (1991) pointed out that persistence of the infection in the Murray et al. deterministic model was due to fractional levels of infected foxes (which he called "atto-foxes") remaining in the population after the primary wave passed. These "atto-foxes" were sufficient to reseed the population and produce the secondary waves observed by Murray et al. (1986) in their model. Mollison pointed out that such a secondary wave would be extremely unlikely to occur in a stochastic setting; rather, repeated disease fade-outs would be the norm. This serves as a clear warning of the dangers of the indiscriminate use of deterministic models, particularly in spatial settings where the population sizes in local settings will be small.

Both the spatial and nonspatial reaction-diffusion models have also been used to assess the impact of various control strategies. Control of infection can be achieved by reducing the density of susceptibles so that the effective reproductive number falls below one; if this happens and is maintained over time, the infectious individuals are unable to replace themselves and so they reduce in number and eventually the disease dies out. In the case of rabies, two primary control strategies have been examined using epidemic models: culling (reducing the population size by killing foxes) and vaccination (achieved by introducing vaccine-doped food into some area) (Anderson et al., 1981; Murray et al., 1986). Both control measures act to reduce the density of susceptibles, but the models clearly show that disease control may be easier to achieve using vaccination rather than culling since the fox population density has a degree of self-regulation. The population dynamics of foxes tends to maintain the total fox density close to the carrying capacity. Removal of foxes by culling, therefore, tends to increase the survival and reproductive chances of the remaining foxes, counteracting the effect of culling. It is also possible that foxes from nonculled neighboring regions could migrate into the habitat opened up by the culling strategy. Vaccination, on the other hand, converts susceptible foxes into immune foxes, more effectively reducing the size of the susceptible population.

As discussed at the beginning of this chapter, the local nature of disease transmission can be used to aid control in situations in which infection is spatially confined in some way. Ring vaccination (or culling) involves reducing the susceptible population in the area neighboring the infection region. Concentration of effort in this way can considerably enhance the probability of eradication, compared to the homogeneous application of control measures. Murray et al. (1986) suggested that a reasonable strategy might be to implement barrier control, where the susceptible density would be reduced in front of the advancing epidemic wave, and they provided analytic calculations of the required width of such a barrier region.

Murray et al. relied on deterministic models in forming their rec-

ommendations for control, and this has led to several criticisms of the
models (although the original authors noted these limitations). In
addition, van den Bosch et al. (1990) criticize some of the assumptions made concerning the movement of foxes. In particular, Murray
et al. assumed that rabid foxes have a higher rate of movement than
nonrabid (i.e., susceptible and latently infected) foxes, an assumption
that, according to van den Bosch et al., is at variance with the results
of several studies.

Interestingly, while the models of Murray et al. (1986) and van den
Bosch et al. (1990) made roughly similar predictions for the functional
relationship between wave speed and the basic reproductive number,
they made quite different predictions regarding the variation in wave
speed with the carrying capacity of the fox population, K. Murray
and colleagues suggested that wave speed is a monotonically increasing function of K; van den Bosch and colleagues showed that speed
first increases, then exhibits a moderate decrease with increasing K.
To a good approximation, the wave speed in the latter model shows
a rapid increase as K passes through a threshold density, but then
remains fairly constant. This behavior was claimed to be in better
agreement with field-based studies that show that the speed of rabies
spread has only a weak dependence on fox population density.

Mollison (1991) compared the use of these two models and discussed
many of the problems that arise when one wants to fit such models
to real-world data in an attempt, for instance, to decide which model
provides a better description of reality. Many of these problems are
issues common to the use of all population models, not just spatial
models — the difficulties in estimating population dynamic parameters have long been noted in the ecological literature. In addition,
given the dependence of the wave speed on the basic reproductive
number, its dependence on population density is an important factor.
This question is one that remains largely unresolved in the general epidemiological literature. Wave speed also depends on the time course
of infection, which is often poorly characterized. For spatial models, the distribution of infectious individuals across space must also
be described. A particular problem here is that wave speeds can be
highly dependent on the tails of the dispersal distribution of infectious
individuals, but since the long-distance interactions that characterize
these tails represent relatively infrequent events, this part of the distribution is least likely to be well characterized. Mollison also includes
an interesting discussion on the relationship between dispersal and the
carrying capacity of the fox population.

It is important to realize that, particularly when several parameters must be fitted from the data set at hand (rather than estimated from independent sources of data), many models are sufficiently flexible that they will be able to fit a given data set quite well. Given the often sparse available data, it is often very difficult to differentiate between the fit provided by two different models. Even if one model provides a better fit, the number of free parameters must be borne in mind: with additional parameters, it becomes much easier to tune the behavior of a model to fit the data. In some cases, a model may make a prediction that is strikingly incorrect (for example, it may make a qualitatively incorrect prediction regarding the direction of change as a certain parameter is varied). In such a situation, the model can clearly be rejected as inadequate. In general, however, such examples are rare and we strongly caution against taking claims of models being in good agreement with data as being correct without keeping the preceding limitations in mind.

4.4.2   The reproduction and dispersal kernel formulation

The reproduction and dispersal kernel formulation is a more general version of the spatially continuous model that specifically allows for nonlocal transmission. Such an approach is of significant use when considering the spread of a human disease under modern conditions where individuals can travel over long distances in a very short time. In general, the use of this approach involves some fairly complex mathematical analysis, and studies using such formulations are often theoretical in nature. Because of this, a full description of the approach is beyond the scope of this book, but it is being used increasingly in studies of the spatial spread of infectious diseases, so we present a brief introduction to such models and the kinds of questions they are being used to address. Readers interested in more details are encouraged to consult Diekmann (1978); Mollison (1991), and van den Bosch et al. (1990).

In the reproduction and dispersal kernel formulation the local rate at which new infections arise, $\partial I(\mathbf{x}, t)/\partial t$, is allowed to depend on the local density of susceptibles and a weighted sum (integral) of the density of infectious individuals elsewhere. These weights are described by a kernel function

$$\frac{\partial I}{\partial t}(\mathbf{x}, t) = S(\mathbf{x}, t) \int \int K(\mathbf{x}, \mathbf{y}, \tau) \frac{\partial I}{\partial t}(\mathbf{y}, t - \tau) \, d\tau d\mathbf{y}. \qquad (4.8)$$

The term $K(\mathbf{x}, \mathbf{y}, \tau)$ describes the rate at which an individual located at point $\mathbf{y}$ who was infected τ time units ago infects susceptible individuals located at point **x**. This formulation, with its dependence on the time since infection, also allows for a general description of the time course of infection.

For many kinds of epidemiological applications it is assumed that the transmission process depends only on the distance between individuals. Thus, the spatial dependence of the kernel function K considers only the magnitude of the distance between individuals, $|\mathbf{x} - \mathbf{y}|$, not the specific locations **x** and **y** or their directional position in space. Under these conditions the speed of spread depends on the shape of the kernel function. In particular, substantial weight in the tails of the kernel (meaning that long-range transmission events are not too unusual) enhance the spatial spread of a disease. If long-range transmission events are relatively infrequent, however, then a stochastic formulation may be necessary in order to adequately capture disease dynamics.

This kind of framework can also be extended to consider a situation where there may be a preferred direction of transmission, such as might be the case when there is airborne transmission of an infectious disease. In such a case one would transform the model to a coordinate frame that moves in the preferred direction. It is also possible to use this framework to model a situation where diffusion occurs at different speeds in different directions. See van den Bosch et al. (1990) for examples of these generalizations of the basic reproduction and dispersal kernel formulation.

4.4.3 Spatial moment equations

The deterministic reaction-diffusion (Equations 4.5 and 4.6) and reproduction and dispersal (Equation 4.8) formulations model just the average behavior of the epidemiological system and ignore stochastic effects. As many previous discussions indicate, however, random effects are often likely to play an important dynamical role in the development of an epidemic. It is therefore desirable to have analytic techniques that can be used to study the impact of stochasticity. Such methods reduce the need for large-scale numerical simulation and are much more likely to give insight into the way in which randomness affects a system.

An alternative approach for the analysis of diffusion or dispersal models involves a description of the moments of the spatial distribution of the population (Bartlett, 1954, 1956, 1960b; Bolker and Pacala, 1997; Daniels, 1977; Lewis, 2000; Lewis and Pacala, 2000). These moments represent averages (or, for second-order moments, variances and covariances) of the distribution of the population taken over a collection of realizations of the underlying stochastic process. Recall that this technique was briefly described in Section 2.4.3.4 when discussing the impact of stochasticity on the basic SIR model.

Many of the studies that have used this approach have been set within an ecological context (Bolker and Pacala, 1997), and invasion behavior has been of particular interest (Lewis, 2000; Lewis and Pacala, 2000). Because there are strong analogies between ecological and epidemiological invasion theory, these invasion studies are of particular relevance to the dynamics of infectious disease.

Invasion processes can often be described extremely well by linear models. As such models are much more amenable to analysis than nonlinear models, their analysis, together with issues surrounding invasion, have tended to dominate the literature. In the stochastic setting, linearity means that the moment equations are decoupled — the equation describing the time evolution of the moments of nth order only involves terms of order n and below. This means, for example, that the equation for the mean only includes terms depending on the mean, and the equation for the second-order moments involves only the second-order moments and the mean.

Lewis and Pacala (2000) presented a particularly detailed analysis of a discrete time stochastic model for the invasion of a population, focusing on the spatial correlations that develop over time. Two questions of particular interest that were addressed are whether this correlation structure approaches some unchanging form (dubbed a "permanence of form" in the correlation structure) and the degree to which the invasion exhibits a patchy structure. The analysis confirmed a result found in other analyses of stochastic spatial models — that the wave speed in stochastic nonlinear settings is strictly less than that predicted by the more common linear analysis of deterministic models.

Although the analyses of Lewis et al. focus on population dynamic models in higher organisms, they have clear implications for epidemiological situations. They highlight the importance of the tails of the dispersal kernel, showing that infrequent long-range disease transmission events can have a major impact not only on the speed at which a disease moves through some region, but also on the degree to which incidence is likely to either show isolated clusters or exhibit a more general, regular, pattern of spread.

The concepts presented in this chapter are well illustrated in applications to the spatial spread of human infectious diseases. We have already discussed the use of metapopulation models in studies of the spread of influenza. In the next chapter we focus on measles, with particular attention paid to how mathematical models are aiding in the attempt to understand the underlying reasons for the long-term cycling of measles and other common childhood diseases. As in the chapter on influenza, our emphasis will be on the kinds of questions addressed and the results of the modeling efforts rather than on the mathematical details. Nonetheless, many of the concepts covered in this chapter will be brought up again in the specific context of measles, particularly concepts relating to cycling, persistence, synchrony, and hierarchical transmission.

Chapter Five

Spatial Heterogeneity and Endemicity: The Case of Measles

Measles has probably been the focus of more geographically oriented modeling work than any other infectious disease and this work has a very long history. Many of the earliest measles modeling studies were stimulated by the mid-19th-century contributions of Peter Ludwig Panum, a Danish physician sent in 1846 to study an outbreak of measles on the Faroe Islands in the North Sea (see Figure 5.1). Panum's detailed 70-page report on the outbreak (Panum, 1847) is often considered to be the first rigorous epidemiological study of the transmission and spread of measles across a landscape. This remarkable report has been translated and reprinted in Panum (1939) and describes not only the levels of morbidity and mortality from measles for different age groups, but also climatic, dietetic, and hygienic conditions prevalent on the islands at the time of the epidemic, presence (or absence) of other common diseases on the islands, detailed discussions of the biology of measles, and observations and conclusions about how and when measles entered particular communities and spread to others on the islands.

Much of the recent work on the geography of measles has focused on understanding how spatial and population characteristics have influenced the development and maintenance of long-term cycles in the incidence of the disease. Cliff et al. (1981) suggest that a disease data set should satisfy four basic requirements in order to be useful for studying the disease in a spatial context. These requirements are

1) Replicability — the disease in question should present a pattern that repeats itself on a regular basis (with each event termed an epidemic wave) so that it can be studied over a significant time period.

2) Stability over time and space — characteristics of the epidemic wave must be consistent in different places and at different times.

3) Observability — the process must be observable both in princi-

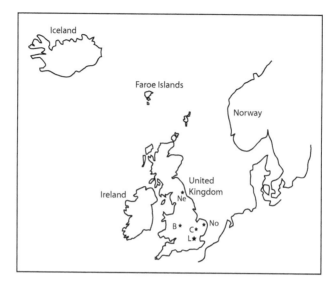

Figure 5.1 Map of countries bordering the North Sea showing cities and countries
discussed in the text. B = Birmingham, C = Cambridge, L = London,
Ne = Newcastle, No = Norwich.

ple and in practice, which requires that observations of the process occur frequently enough to allow several individual waves
to be distinguished.

4) Isolation — the individual waves need to be separated in time
and space, as too much overlap will make observed patterns too
complex.

The symptoms of measles are quite marked, so it is easily diagnosed.
Consequently, reasonably accurate incidence data for the disease have
been routinely collected in Western Europe and North America for
over a century, providing a long enough time span to be able to identify
temporal patterns. In addition, the measles virus is highly stable evo-
lutionarily, which makes it reasonable to assume that a population's
experience with the disease over long time spans has been relatively
stable as well.

Observations of the long-term incidence rates of measles show that
these data do, in fact, fulfill Cliff et al.'s basic requirements. As
Figures 5.2a-c show, when populations are large, the disease cycles
regularly over long periods of time. As illustrated by Figure 5.2d,

however, cycling is less apparent when populations are small because under those conditions the disease dies out between epidemics and does not flare up without re-introduction from outside the population. Figures 5.2a-d also show that the epidemic waves are similar from place to place and over time, although the introduction of widespread vaccination in the mid-1960s led to qualitative changes in the length and amplitude of observed cycles. The requirement of observability of measles is fulfilled by the nature of the virus, its ease of diagnosis, and the propensity for record keeping in Western Europe and North America. And as Figure 5.2 shows, individual waves are clearly separated in time and space, fulfilling the criterion of isolation.

Research on the geography of measles has followed two major directions: 1) understanding the underlying causes of the long-term persistence and regular cycling of the disease, and 2) understanding the nature of patterns of spread of the disease across space and time. The vast majority of the modeling and geographic literature on both of these issues is centered around very high-quality data sets and exemplary use of those data within a modeling framework. Until recently the main spatially focused questions of interest to mathematical modelers centered on understanding how spatial heterogeneity (i.e., variability over space in disease incidence) could help to explain maintenance of the disease over time within different populations, while the study of spatial spread was largely limited to geographers using predominantly statistical techniques. In recent years, however, mathematical modelers have devoted more attention to explaining how the disease spreads between communities across time and space. A major reason for this shift is the growing recognition that, as has been discussed in previous chapters, links between communities can help to prevent fadeouts within them, thereby enabling a disease to persist. Consequently, many of the models that were originally developed to address spatial heterogeneity and disease persistence are also being used to consider the question of spatial coupling and spatial spread between communities.

Measles is an acute, highly communicable viral disease that, prior to the availability of immunizations, affected almost all children. Historically it was among the most serious of childhood illnesses, especially in malnourished children. Transmission of the virus occurs through airborne droplet spread and through contact with nasal or throat secretions of infectious individuals. Figure 5.3 shows the progression of the disease in an infected individual, a pattern that was recognized and documented by Panum in his classic 1847 monograph (Panum, 1847, 1939). Upon infection, a person enters an incubation stage of

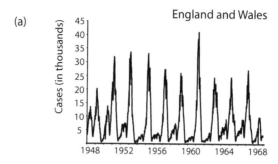

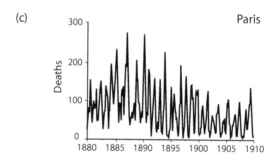

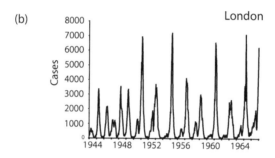

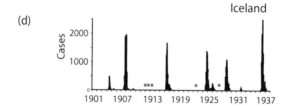

Figure 5.2 Time series of measles incidence in different sized cities and regions. a) Cases reported per week in England and Wales. b) Bi-weekly cases in London. c) Deaths per month in Paris [redrawn from Anderson et al. (1984), Figure 1d]. d) Monthly cases in Iceland [redrawn from Cliff and Haggett (1983)]. Stars on the Iceland graph indicate years with sporadic cases.

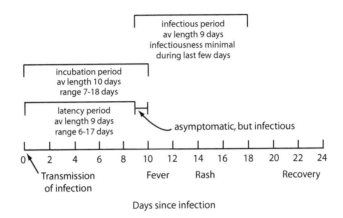

Figure 5.3 The progression of a measles infection.

approximately 10 days until the onset of fever, with the characteristic rash appearing about 4 days later. An infected person is infectious from slightly before the beginning of the prodromal stage until about 4 days after the appearance of the rash, although infectiousness declines significantly after the second day of the rash (Heymann, 2004). The clinical features of the disease are so marked that it can be recognized in the earliest historical records. It is thought that the disease dates to human prehistory (Cliff et al., 1993), perhaps originating in association with the domestication of animals and the corresponding rise in human settlement size (Cockburn, 1971; Fiennes, 1978).

Because of the contagiousness of the disease, a significant number of births must occur yearly in order to maintain a susceptible population large enough to continue the chain of infections and prevent die outs in a population. Bartlett (1957, 1960a) used mathematical analysis and analysis of prevalence data in different sized populations to estimate the critical community size needed to maintain the disease in an endemic state. His studies suggested that unless a population consists of around 300-500,000 people, the number of annual births will be too small to maintain the disease. One of the criticisms of Bartlett's analysis, however, is that the populations he used in his analyses were not closed to migration, so that it is not clear how well his estimate reflected the actual critical community size. To address this issue,

Black (1966) used a similar approach with data from a series of island populations, which were more isolated than the cities Bartlett used and therefore were not subject to the same kinds of criticisms. His results showed that the critical community size for island populations was of the same order of magnitude, providing strong support for Bartlett's general conclusion. Essentially what Bartlett's and Black's results imply is that in populations larger than the critical community size, cases of the disease would always be apparent (i.e., the disease would be endemic), although there would also be periodic epidemics that were more widespread. In populations below this size, epidemics would be followed by stretches of time with no reported cases until the disease was reintroduced from outside, upon which there would be a new epidemic. The development of mathematical models that would explain how such patterns could be maintained and predicted within a region has been one of the major activities of spatial measles modeling.

5.1 THE PERSISTENCE AND LONG-TERM CYCLING OF MEASLES

Work on understanding how spatial heterogeneity has affected the long-term persistence and cycling of measles epidemics was stimulated by analyses of a long time series of weekly case reports of measles between 1948 and 1966 in England and Wales (see Figure 5.2a), which clearly showed regular two-year cycles of the disease throughout the time period. In addition to this data set, data at the city level in England and Wales and from New York City, Baltimore, Copenhagen, and several other locations have been analyzed in association with mathematical models, and the time periods involved have been extended to include the years after the introduction of widespread vaccination in the mid-1960s. The impact of this practice was significant — changing the pattern in most places from one of biennial highly regular cycles to one of annual, less regular cycles.

   The use of models to help explain features of the measles time series from western Europe and North America has a very long history, beginning with the classic works of Hamer (1906), Soper (1929), Wilson and Worcester (1945a), Bartlett (1956, 1957), and London and Yorke (1973). Building upon this body of research, a number of more recent models have been developed and analyzed. These models address several overlapping questions related to measles epidemiology. In this section we discuss how models without spatial spread have been used to explore the underlying factors responsible for the long-term persistence and cycling of the disease. In the next section we focus on models used to help understand the relationship between long-term persistence and cycling and the synchronization of epidemics in a spatial context, and how those models aid in understanding the long-term patterns of spread of the disease across time and space.

A variety of models have been used to help in understanding why the incidence of measles exhibits such regular and long-standing cycles in large cities of the United States and western Europe, while in smaller populations the cycles are either less regular or absent. Most of the earliest models (e.g., Bartlett, 1957; Hamer, 1906; Soper, 1929) focused on understanding the situation in large cities, and they assumed a constant rate of transmission. Although they were able to reproduce cycling, the pattern was one of damped oscillations converging to a fixed equilibrium rather than the sustained oscillations observed in actual data (Bailey, 1975). In an attempt to remedy this, London and Yorke (1973) and Fine and Clarkson (1982) incorporated seasonally varying contact rates into their models. These models were able to keep oscillations from dying out, but they were still unable to reproduce the existing patterns adequately.

Another relatively early approach to explaining the observed large city data patterns involved the use of chaos theory (e.g., Olsen et al., 1988; Schaffer, 1985; Schaffer and Kot, 1985). These models were able to approximate the oscillatory behavior observed in the large cities, but they required extreme and unrealistic levels of seasonal forcing in order to do so, and they also did not reproduce the observed patterns of extinction of epidemics in different communities (commonly referred to as fadeout) (Bolker and Grenfell, 1995; Grenfell, 1992).

A third relatively early approach was that of Schenzle (1984), who combined seasonal forcing with age structuring so that he could capture the effects on epidemic patterns of differences in school calendars and mixing among children of different ages. This model, known as the realistic age structure (RAS) model, clearly illustrated the importance of school-related seasonal forcing, and many more recent models addressing the persistence and regional spread of measles are based on this framework. Although the RAS model worked very well for the England and Wales data, it could not reproduce the more complex patterns observed in other cities, however (Bolker and Grenfell, 1993). In addition, the RAS model and the other early models predicted critical community sizes that were much greater than the 300-500,000 threshold determined by Bartlett (1957, 1960a) and Black (1966).

During the 1990s a number of refinements of these models were made and additional studies focused on reproducing observed oscillations, the pattern of fadeout, and realistic critical community sizes. The models included a stochastic SEIR model (Grenfell, 1992), a cross-coupled metapopulation stochastic RAS model (Bolker and Grenfell, 1993, 1995), a RAS model with yearly age classes through age five (Ferguson et al., 1996), a RAS model with nonconstant incubation and infection periods (Keeling and Grenfell, 1997, 1998), and a semi-mechanistic model that combined a seasonally forced SEIR model with a statistical time series approach (Ellner et al., 1998a). In general, these models improved the fit between model oscillations and the real data, but they still estimated critical community sizes that were too large and they still were unable to adequately reproduce the fadeout patterns.

The most recent model used to help in understanding western European and North American measles time series data is the TSIR model proposed by Bjørnstad et al. (2002); Finkenstädt and Grenfell (2000), and Grenfell et al. (2002). This model builds on the idea of Ellner et al. (1998a) to combine a dynamic mathematical approach with a statistical time series approach (TSIR stands for "time series - susceptible - infected - recovered"). Results of analyses of this model suggest that the endemicity of measles in large cities is related both to seasonally varying contact rates and to longer-term variations in birth rate. In addition, results support a common hypothesis suggested by many researchers that the epidemic experience of communities smaller than Bartlett's critical community size is largely related to the joint effects of demographic stochasticity and pathogen extinction/reintroduction. This latter hypothesis was also supported by Rhodes and Anderson (1996), who used a lattice-based SEIR model to study the spread of measles in the small and isolated population of the Faroe Islands.

Before turning to models that address issues of spatial structure, one other body of work deserves mention. In a slight variation of all this work, Rohani and colleagues examined the ability of deterministic and stochastic seasonally forced SEIR models to predict oscillatory behavior of pertussis as well as measles, both by looking at the pathogens individually and by considering them simultaneously (Rohani et al., 1998, 1999, 2002, 2003). They found that although deterministic models could be used to study many measles-related questions, a stochastic framework was absolutely necessary for studies of pertussis dynamics. (A similar conclusion was reached by Hethcote (1998).) In addition to the need for stochastic models, Rohani and colleagues showed that pertussis and measles exhibited opposite patterns of synchrony (discussed further below), and, furthermore, when both pathogens were considered together in a model, the dynamical behavior was completely different from that observed in models considering either pathogen alone (Rohani et al., 2003). These models clearly point out the importance of carefully considering the biological characteristics of different pathogens when devising models for their transmission and spread and attest to the potential pitfalls of assuming that a particular pathogen affects its host independently of the effects of any other pathogens present. Nonetheless, consideration of the joint effects of co-circulating pathogens introduces an additional level of complexity that may be undesirable, depending on the nature of the questions being addressed.

5.2   SPATIAL HETEROGENEITY, SYNCHRONY, AND THE SPATIAL SPREAD OF MEASLES

Most of the models discussed in the previous section either consider one large, homogeneous population or consider an age-structured population, but do not take the spatial structure of the populations into account. In thinking about the issue of fadeout, however, researchers began to recognize that a consideration of spatial structure might help explain fadeout, primarily because contact between groups could facilitate pathogen spread from subpopulations experiencing a disease outbreak to disease-free subpopulations. Some degree of spatial structure was incorporated into measles models sporadically until the mid-1980s (e.g., Bartlett, 1956; Murray and Cliff, 1977); consideration of the importance of spatial structure became especially prominent in measles models of the 1990s and later.

Almost all of the earliest models incorporating spatial structure focused on determining the role of spatial heterogeneity in the persistence or extinction of measles within and among communities. In other words, the focus of these models was on determining how the coupling among communities could facilitate or prohibit the maintenance of an epidemic within each community and across an entire region. One feature of such spatial systems that proved to be of considerable importance in determining whether a disease could persist in a community or region is whether outbreaks in neighboring communities were synchronized with each other or were out of phase. Recall from the previous chapter that asynchrony between communities can provide opportunities for the reintroduction of pathogens after local extinction, while synchronized epidemics tend to fade out simultaneously, leading to wider regional extinction. The issue of synchrony was thus a natural focus for early spatially structured models. For the most part, however, aside from the occasional study (e.g., Murray and Cliff, 1977), questions of how the disease spread across time and space from one community to another within a region were not considered in these early models.

During the early to mid-1980s mathematical modelers spent much effort exploring the effectiveness of different potential immunization strategies for a variety of human viral diseases, including measles, rubella, and pertussis. Most of these incorporated some kind of population structure, with the most common being age structure, but occasionally some type of spatial structure was considered (although the spatial models usually did not include age structure). The model of Hethcote and Van Ark (1987) and the similar "cities and villages" model of May and Anderson (1984) are examples of early spatially structured models designed to evaluate immunization programs.

Work addressing the impact of spatial structure on pathogen persistence began in earnest in the early to mid-1990s. For example, Grenfell (1992) assumed a simple spatial arrangement in which a model city of one million inhabitants was divided equally into two halves. He then considered the effect of different degrees of coupling between the two halves, ranging from no coupling to complete coupling. Results showed that simply including spatial coupling was not sufficient to realistically characterize the observed patterns. Lloyd and May (1996) and Lloyd and Jansen (2004) analyzed a seasonally forced spatial model with n subpopulations to look at the relationship between coupling between subpopulations and synchronization of epidemic oscillations across subpopulations. The model did not include explicit movement between cities, but did allow contact between individuals from different cities. Analysis of this model showed that the seasonally forced spatial model led to more complex behavior and was able to predict critical community size better than the nonspatial, but seasonally forced model. In addition, unless the coupling between communities was very weak, epidemics in different communities within a region tended to become synchronized with one another.

Bolker and Grenfell (1995) added a metapopulation structure to the more complicated RAS model that included age structure and seasonal forcing. Their model also suggested that the addition of spatial structure could enhance the persistence of a disease. Their results helped to explain fadeout behavior, although the model was still unable to reduce the predicted critical community size to observed levels (Grenfell and Harwood, 1997).

Building upon both their 1995 paper and the earlier work of May and Anderson (1984), Grenfell and Bolker (1998) showed that fadeout appears to be mostly a population size effect rather than an urban-rural effect — urban and rural communities of comparable size experienced similar risks for fadeout of epidemics. Grenfell et al. (2001) used several different spatially coupled models to home in on the way that population size influenced fadeout and synchrony. Consistent with the theoretical results of Lloyd and May (1996) and Lloyd and Jansen (2004), analysis of these models showed that the strong coupling between large cities generated highly synchronized epidemics while communities that were more weakly coupled moved away from synchrony with the larger centers.

Most of the studies of synchrony of measles epidemics across communities involve local analyses of the systems and so they cannot show for certain whether a system will synchronize; rather they show only that the system either cannot synchronize or that it might synchronize (although the probability of the latter event could be vanishingly small) (Earn, personal communication). Earn et al. (2000a) performed global analyses to identify conditions under which populations would or would not develop synchronous oscillations. Results of these analyses are discussed with reference to two questions. First, how can conservation corridors be maintained in order to prevent synchrony of different subpopulations of endangered species and the extinction that might follow such synchrony? Second, how can synchrony be promoted in order to increase the chance of eradicating an infectious disease? Earn and Levin (2006) built on this work and proved a global theorem that provided insight into the conditions necessary to guarantee that a system would synchronize.

One of the primary factors influencing persistence of measles at the regional level is undoubtedly the fact that there are constant social interactions among people from different communities within a region. These interactions ensure that, even if a disease dies out within a community it can be reintroduced fairly quickly, thereby maintaining the presence of the disease within the region. As mentioned above, this spatial coupling between communities as a consequence of the social interactions has been incorporated into at least some of the models that focus on understanding spatial heterogeneity. However, the social interactions between communities serve another purpose — they allow the disease to spread across both time and space. These patterns of spread are most observable when considering a single epidemic, but they can also be evaluated over a longer period of time.

Studies looking at the spatial spread of measles are not as common as those attempting to explain long-term persistence across space. The majority of models used in this task employ a cross-coupling framework that considers only the contact between communities or regions, but does not explicitly model the process by which that contact comes about. Notable exceptions to this include the studies of Murray and Cliff (1977) and Xia et al. (2004) (discussed further below), both of which modeled the interaction between communities with a gravity model (i.e., the strength of the connection between two locations is a function of the distance between the locations and their relative sizes).

Finkenstädt and Grenfell (1998) used a generalized linear model with cross-coupling between cities to investigate the influence of local and regional effects in determining epidemic patterns. Because of a lack of data on actual contact patterns among locations, they used a range of indirect measures that were based on the distance between communities and regional population density. They found that the dynamics of major epidemics were dominated by local deterministic population dynamics, but that minor epidemics and associated fadeouts were affected by both population dynamics and regional geographical structure. Grenfell et al. (2001) used wavelet phase analysis and the TSIR epidemic model to demonstrate the existence of recurrent epidemic traveling waves in the England and Wales measles data set. These waves moved regionally from large cities to small towns in a hierarchical fashion. They also analyzed how the spatial waves were related to the type of coupling between communities and found that hierarchical waves, such as those they observed, would arise when a group of small towns surrounded a large population center. The presence of multiple large centers may lead to more complicated regional patterns, however, in which some areas may not be synchronized with the predominant large center because of the draw of secondary large centers. Grenfell et al. (2001) hypothesize that this behavior may help explain why Norwich was not synchronized with the rest of England over a 16-year period, unlike the relatively close city of Cambridge (Figure 5.4; see also Figure 1 in He and Stone (2003) and see Figure 5.1 for locations of these cities). (Note, however, that Cambridge and Norwich become more synchronized after 1960.)

Two recent models have been used in attempts to explain the lack of synchronization observed by Grenfell et al. (2001). As mentioned above, Xia et al. (2004) added a gravity model to the TSIR model. They considered a population of 5 million inhabitants surrounded by 500 satellites of 100,000 people each. Results of the analysis of this model showed that the movement of individuals did not affect the

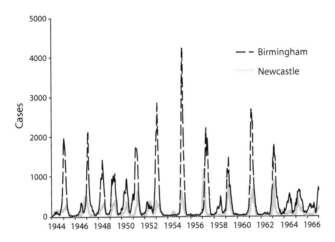

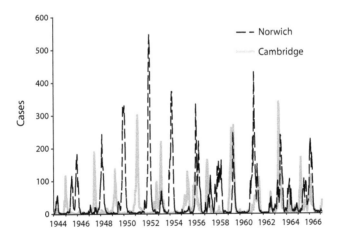

Figure 5.4 Synchronization of measles in four British cities. Data are reported biweekly.

core population dynamics much because the number of locally produced infectious individuals in the large population center was much
larger than the number of infected travelers carrying the disease in
from outside. Consistent with the results of Grenfell et al. (2001),
simulations of the TSIR+gravity model indicated that communities
close to the core city were highly synchronized with that city, while
those further away (and more weakly coupled) were less synchronized.
Furthermore, peripheral communities tended to exhibit irregular epidemics with long disease-free periods, much like the patterns observed
in actual time series from small, isolated communities. These and
other results indicate that this model is successful in predicting the
general patterns observed in the spatiotemporal dynamics of measles,
although the fadeout behavior is still not quite realistic and the results
depend critically on the parameters of the gravity term. The model
is also unable to explain the anomaly of Cambridge and Norwich observed by Grenfell et al. (2001).

In a slight variant of other models, He and Stone (2003) used a
discrete time formulation of the classic SIR model, with the addition of
temporary immunity so that individuals could return to a susceptible
state after sufficient time passed (often called the "SIRS" model).
They chose this model because it has a known propensity to oscillate
(Cooke et al., 1977; Girvan et al., 2002; Kuperman and Abramson,
2001) and can therefore capture the essential dynamics of measles, but
is reasonably tractable analytically. Their results are similar to those
of Grenfell et al. (2001), even though the latter model was seasonally
forced. Their results also provide strong support for the suggestions
made by Grenfell et al. (2001) that the draw of secondary large centers
may influence epidemic synchronization patterns within a region.

The vast majority of insights about the underlying factors influencing spatial patterns of measles have been derived from models analyzing long-term incidence patterns from western Europe, particularly
England and Wales, and occasionally from the United States. Recent
studies have indicated, however, that the kinds of results observed
for the United States and western Europe may not be fully generalizable to other parts of the world. In particular, Ferrari et al. (2008)
considered the dynamics of measles in the sub-Saharan country of
Niger. Measles transmission in this country is highly seasonal, with
outbreaks coinciding with the end of the annual rainy season. Analyses of outbreaks in this country indicate that the high seasonality
results in more irregular dynamics than predicted by models based
on western European historical data. These irregular dynamics have
strong implications for the development of effective vaccination and

other control strategies. Furthermore, it is clear from this work that there is a need for caution when transferring insights and control strategies chosen on the basis of those insights from the populations from which they are derived to new situations.

The most significant body of work looking at how measles actually spreads across space and time is the work of Cliff, Haggett, and colleagues on the spread of measles in Iceland (see Figure 5.1). This work is a groundbreaking body of research looking specifically at how to describe, measure, and predict patterns of geographic spread of infectious diseases. It has been the focus of two major books (Cliff et al., 1981, 1993) as well as several scholarly articles (e.g., Cliff and Haggett, 1980, 1983; Cliff et al., 1983a,b; Cliff and Haggett, 1984; Cliff and Ord, 1985; Cliff and Haggett, 1993). The majority of this work has drawn upon primarily statistical techniques that are discussed in more detail in Chapter 8. These techniques have generated a detailed description and analysis of patterns of spread of measles among communities on Iceland from the late 1800s through the first three-quarters of the 1900s.

The terrain of Iceland is very rugged, and the interior of the island has an especially harsh climate. Consequently, the majority of the population lives in coastal communities that are interspersed with inlets and fjords, limiting the extent of between community interactions. Demographic records show that between 1896 and 1975 there were 16 distinct waves of measles. Typically the waves lasted about a year and a half and reached over 40 of the 50 medical districts on the island. Figure 5.5 shows the timing and extent of a 1916-17 measles epidemic on the island. Between waves the island would experience an average of about three years with no cases of the disease (Cliff and Haggett, 1984). Using detailed medical records, Cliff and colleagues were able to reconstruct not only the patterns of spread among regions within the island for any given epidemic, but also the probable sources on the European mainland for many of the 16 observed epidemic waves. They also identified three primary factors that underlay many of the observed patterns: 1) the mobility of the index case, 2) the contribution of communal activities such as local gatherings, and 3) the countermeasures implemented to try to control epidemics.

Information on patterns of spread of measles throughout Iceland and other results from the analyses of Cliff and colleagues were used to develop forecasting models to predict the future spread of infectious diseases on the island (Cliff et al., 1981, 1993; Cliff and Ord, 1985). Results of their forecasting models were mixed, with a logistic regression model performing the best (Cliff and Ord, 1985), but that

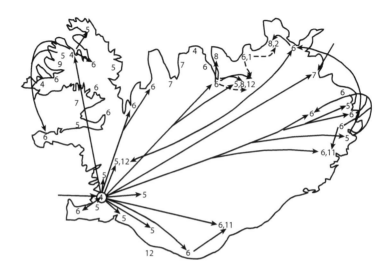

Figure 5.5 Spread of the 1916-17 measles epidemic on Iceland. Numbers refer to month of the year when cases were first recorded in a particular district. Adapted from Cliff et al. (1981), Figure 4.5.

model was still unable to capture all the details of observed epidemics.

In addition to the Iceland work, Cliff and colleagues studied the spread of measles in Fiji and the Pacific, the northeastern United States, and a few other regions. Their Fiji and Pacific study (Cliff and Haggett, 1985) was primarily descriptive, with some spatial autocorrelation analysis. Studies of the spread of measles in the northeastern United States focused on identifying the spatial structure of reported measles morbidity over a 27-year period (Cliff et al., 1992a, 1995) and on measuring the degree to which the behavior of a time series in one region was correlated to that in another region. Cliff and colleagues also investigated whether the correlations held at different geographic scales (Cliff et al., 1992b), although they did not consider the spatial spread of measles. Results of these studies indicated that the incidence of measles was dominated by local effects — states in geographic proximity tended to be most highly correlated with one another, and this pattern was retained well after the introduction of widespread vacination.

Finally, in an early modeling study of the spatial spread of measles, Murray and Cliff (1977) developed a multiregional stochastic compartmental epidemic model and simulated measles spread among and within General Register Office areas (local health authority reporting units) of the city of Bristol. Their results suggested that a homogeneous mixing assumption within areas would not reflect observed patterns well unless the areas were of small to moderate size. This led them to recommend that analysis of data from larger cities, such as Bristol, be broken down into smaller units if possible.

The work of Cliff and colleagues and of Grenfell and others on describing and explaining the role of space in generating patterns of measles disease transmission within and among communities is unparalleled and clearly provides an excellent example of how epidemics can be studied within a spatial framework. Because of this emphasis, much is known and understood about how and why measles varies across space and spreads across space and time. In addition, much of the knowledge derived from the study of measles helps in understanding the persistence and spread of many other diseases. Nonetheless, both bodies of research also clearly indicate that we do not yet fully understand all the reasons for the observed long-term cycling of measles and many other diseases, not only in western Europe and North America where there are high-quality data sets extending over many decades, but also (and especially) in less developed regions of the world where data are less adequate and studies are limited.

Chapter Six

Modeling Geographic Spread II:

Individual-based Approaches

Epidemiologists have long had a standard procedure, contact tracing, that they have followed in trying to isolate the cause of a disease outbreak and in attempting to control the outbreak. Contact tracing involves interviewing cases of an infectious disease to determine who they may have come into contact with while infectious, finding the identified contacts and determining whether they also became infected, and, if so, attempting to identify their contacts. The process continues until the all of the new persons traced are uninfected (at least in theory) (Morris, 2004b). Both treatment (and isolation if warranted) of identified cases and implementation of preventive measures to limit further spread of the disease are an integral part of this process.

Contact tracing was an essential component of the public health response to the 2003 SARS outbreak throughout the world. For example, Varia et al. (2003) describe how the SARS outbreak spread in Toronto, Canada, which reported well over 100 cases during the epidemic. The disease was first introduced into Canada by a resident of Toronto who returned home on 23 February 2003 from a visit to Hong Kong. While in Hong Kong, she stayed at a hotel in Kowloon. Later analysis indicated that the hotel in question experienced a cluster of 13 cases, but the Toronto woman did not come down with the illness until after her return to Canada. She then spread the disease to family members. One of these family members was admitted to a local hospital after going to the emergency room, and this person initiated a widespread hospital-based (nosocomial) outbreak. Varia et al. (2003) conducted a detailed analysis of the initial Toronto SARS cases, including both cases in people who became infected in the hospital and those in their contacts outside the hospital. In the course of their study they identified at least 6 generations of infection, including four generations that resulted from nosocomial spread.

Figure 6.1 shows the transmission links ascertained by Varia et al. (2003). It is important to note, however, that these data show only the contacts that actually resulted in infection and are thus a subset of all possible contacts that carried the risk of disease transmission. Because of the way such contacts are identified, the contact tracing methods used by epidemiologists give a biased view of the entire set of contacts linking infectious individuals to others.

Data of the type analyzed by Varia et al. (2003) are commonly observed when looking at person-to-person spread of infectious diseases. Such patterns derive from the social interactions between different individuals within a community and they are effectively described in terms of a graph or network. In the simplest cases, each node on the graph represents an individual member of the population and edges between nodes indicate a social link between the individuals represented by the nodes. In the case of disease transmission, these edges also indicate possible routes by which infection can spread between individuals. Depending on the level at which the population is being modeled, the "individual" could represent some collection of individuals, such as a family, a school, or even an entire community (which is better thought of as a metapopulation, as we described in Chapter 4). Such models do not necessarily include an explicit spatial framework — in many cases the individuals are linked socially and the "space" being modeled is a social space. Sometimes, though, the individuals are situated in geographical space; such models would consider how diseases spread within the area filled by the individuals.

As has been illustrated in many of the applications discussed in this book, in reality the relevant space for disease transmission includes both physical proximity and social proximity and it is not always clear how best to define the spatial dimension of a model. Networks of interaction, which explicitly consider the actual links between individuals regardless of the underlying reasons for those links, implicitly include both physical and social proximity, and are one strategy that is being used increasingly in models for the spread of infectious diseases. In fact, most individual-based approaches to the geographic spread of human diseases are built around some kind of network structure. Thus, our focus in this chapter will be on describing the nature of network approaches and the insights about disease transmission patterns that have been gained from them.

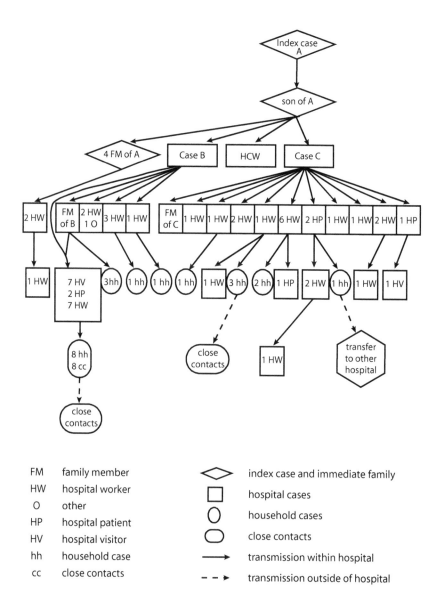

Figure 6.1 A network of SARS cases in Toronto during the 2003 epidemic. Cases
          occurring during the same generation of infection are placed in the same
          row of the figure. Adapted from Varia et al. (2003), Figure 2.

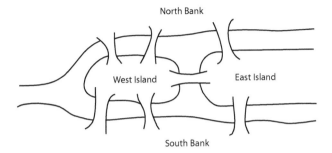

Figure 6.2 Layout of bridges in the town of Königsberg.

6.1 HISTORICAL UNDERPINNINGS OF THE USE OF NETWORKS IN EPIDEMIOLOGY

Network approaches in epidemiology have exploded within the last 10 years or so, and many of these studies are described in this and other chapters. It is important to realize, however, that although applications to epidemiological questions have become common only recently, the use of network approaches to study social interactions and social contact (the mechanism by which directly transmitted diseases spread among humans) has a long history. Such studies have generally been the focus of sociologists, anthropologists, and other social scientists and are intimately connected to an area of mathematics called graph theory.

The roots of the study of graph theory applied to practical human problems are often said to derive from a famous problem, the Königsberg bridge problem, solved by the mathematician Leonhard Euler in 1736. The town of Königsberg, Germany had seven bridges linking the four parts of the town — two islands and the two sides of the river — to each other (see Figure 6.2). Residents of the town wanted to find out if it was possible to walk a circuit through all four parts of the town, crossing each of the seven bridges exactly once. Euler used graph theory to show that such a circuit through Königsberg was impossible.

According to Roberts (1976), early uses of graph theory included applications to electrical networks (Kirchoff, 1847), organic chemistry (Cayley, 1857, 1874), puzzles, and maps and map coloring (a classical graph theory problem that still stimulates many mathematical studies). Applications to the analysis of social interactions began to show up somewhat later, with most researchers giving Harary and Norman (1953) and Harary et al. (1965) credit for introducing the mathematical techniques of graph theory to social scientists (Roberts, 1979).

Roberts (1979) and Newman (2003d) provide an overview of many of the most important early applications of graph theory in the social sciences. A number of early papers in this area have also been reprinted in Leinhardt (1977). Three types of applications are of particular relevance to network models in epidemiology — studies of the overall structure of social networks and how they influence patterns of disease spread through a population, studies of the impact of social cliques or social clusters of individuals on rates and patterns of disease spread, and studies of social status and the relative position of individuals within social structures.

The most important of these for epidemiological studies is the study of social networks, or the patterns of interaction between different individuals within a group. Much of the work in this area has been largely descriptive, but it has led to greater understanding of the characteristics of social interactions and how network conformations may promote or inhibit the spread of such things as pathogens, information, or materials through a population. Moreno (1934) first suggested using a graph to represent the structure of a social network. He let the vertices of his graph represent individuals, and the arcs between vertices signified a social relationship between the two individuals represented by the vertices in question. The resulting diagram was referred to as a sociogram, and through the years many studies have used graph theory to aid in understanding the properties of sociograms (see, for example, Davis and Leinhardt, 1972; Holland and Leinhardt, 1971, 1976; Rapoport, 1957). Some of these properties will be described below, as they have clear impact for understanding how and why diseases spread along networks. Other early studies of the characteristics of social networks, most of which incorporated sociograms, include a study of the social circles of women in a southern U.S. city (Davis et al., 1941), studies of the friendship networks of school children (Fararo and Sunshine, 1989; Rapoport and Horvath, 1961), and a study of the social networks of factory workers in Chicago during the 1930s (Roethlisberger and Dickson, 1939).

A second kind of graph theory application that is of relevance to epidemic spread is the study of the impact of clustering of individuals into social cliques. Early studies of social cliques include Bron and Kerbosch (1973), Granovetter (1973), Heil and White (1976), and Luce (1950). Infectious disease transmission can be intensified within social cliques because of greater opportunities for social contact promoting transmission, and so the size and types of social cliques within a community can have strong effects on patterns of spread throughout the community. Cliques can also reduce the potential for spread — they can result in overlapping neighborhoods that effectively dilute the pool of potential new hosts for an infection because there is an increased number of redundant links to any susceptible individual. As a consequence, a high degree of clustering in a network can lower the epidemic threshold and allow saturation of a population at lower levels of transmission, but it may also reduce the overall number of individuals who become infected (Newman, 2003c).

Graph theory has also been used extensively in studies of social status and the relative positions of different individuals within a social network. Such studies focus extensively on the notion of centrality, a concept that will be discussed further below. According to Roberts (1979), the concept was introduced by Bavelas to describe how easily any particular individual can influence all the other individuals in the group. A variety of other measures have also been devised (see Roberts (1979) for examples of other studies in this area). Sattenspiel et al. (2000) illustrated the importance of centrality of a community in determining patterns of epidemic spread; occupying a central position in a social network plays a similar role at the individual level.

Many other examples of applications of graph theory to the study of social interactions are present in the literature; the papers discussed here are only intended to illustrate the long history of this study. It has become a major area of emphasis in the social sciences, with an entire journal, *Social Networks*, devoted to such studies. Nonetheless, it was not until the late 1980s, when the AIDS epidemic became the focus of disease modeling efforts, that social networks began to play a prominent role in epidemic modeling. Since that time network concepts have been central to understanding the transmission of sexually transmitted infections of all kinds, and, in addition, they are now becoming a more prominent feature of epidemic models for many other diseases. It should be noted, however, that there are many kinds of diseases for which network approaches are not particularly helpful. For example, such models would not work well for many vector-borne diseases because their transmission depends primarily upon a mobile insect or other vector rather than upon direct connections between humans.

6.2   THE NATURE OF NETWORKS

So what exactly are networks and how do they get incorporated into epidemic models? Networks are all around us and include, for example, the internet (an information network), cell phones (a communication network), airline travel (a transportation network), and many other networks that we recognize and understand because of the specialized nature of our brain and nervous system (a neural network). As described above, at their essence networks consist of a number of nodes (or vertices) with edges connecting them. The nodes represent individuals or groups and the edges represent the type of interaction between particular individuals or groups. See Figure 6.3 for examples of how networks can be represented.

Many of the standard network analysis techniques assume a static, or unchanging, network. As discussed in Chapter 2, demographic changes in the population can effectively be ignored for a rapidly spreading infection. In a similar way, it is often assumed that the contact structure of a population remains static over the timescale of a short-lived outbreak. Thus, static network models may provide a good description for infections that spread rapidly through a population, and this is one setting in which network approaches have commonly been applied. Network approaches have also become the standard in models for the transmission of sexually transmitted diseases, where the emphasis is upon partnerships rather than individuals as the primary unit of analysis. This emphasis has revolutionized the study of how sexual behavior influences the transmission of disease (Morris, 2004b).

When attempting to model disease transmission in a particular situation, detailed knowledge of the population at hand is usually necessary in order to enable the construction of a realistic network depicting the population. In most cases, this task is manageable only for small populations. Obtaining a detailed description of the contact structure within a large population requires an enormous effort, and so the instances in which this has been carried out are few (see, for example, Eubank et al., 2004; Potterat et al., 2004).

Within the literature of mathematical epidemiology, network studies have pursued two complementary, but distinct directions. On the one hand, several studies have looked at the impact of network structures on the spread of particular epidemics such as the 1918-19 flu or the AIDS epidemic. On the other hand, conceptual studies typically focus on a particular network, or on a particular class of networks and are designed to explore the consequences of network structure more

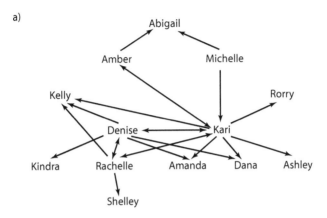

Figure 6.3 Examples of different networks. a) Friendship links among girls in a British elementary school class in 1993. All names are pseudonyms. An arrow pointing to a child indicates that the person at the other end of the arrow said the girl was one of her friends. b) The general structure of a neural network model, a structure that originated after examination of the structure of the central nervous system, but that is now used in a number of different applications.

theoretically rather than trying to provide realistic depictions of real-world populations. For example, even though few populations conform to the rigid description provided by lattice models such as those described below and illustrated in Figure 6.6, such models are used frequently because their interactions are purely local in nature and so they provide a simple characterization of settings in which transmission is mainly (or entirely) local. Because they are more likely to be amenable to mathematical analysis, simple network types such as the lattice model have proved useful in the process of identifying which network properties are of most importance in determining patterns of disease transmission.

Network approaches are an excellent way to describe and understand the nature of social links between individuals and groups at a particular time and place, but problems arise when population characteristics change over time. For example, in order to model births and deaths of individuals, nodes must be added or removed from the network, as must edges between these nodes and their neighbors. Similarly, edges must be rewired in order to model changes in the interactions between individuals, which might occur, for instance, when individuals are allowed to move from place to place. Some of these problems can be ameliorated by adopting a slightly more complex approach that allows nodes to exist in an empty state (see, for example, Keeling, 1999a). In this framework, nodes represent sites that could potentially be occupied by individuals, with the number of nodes, or sites, being greater than the number of individuals in the population. Births are modeled by the insertion of susceptible individuals into empty sites and deaths are modeled by the removal of individuals, leaving empty sites. Random movement of individuals can be built into a lattice model by allowing members of the population to move from their site to a neighboring empty site, in a way that is somewhat akin to the diffusion of the simplest spatially continuous models.

6.3   THE LANGUAGE OF NETWORK ANALYSIS

As with many other specialized areas, network analysis involves a number of unique terms and concepts that may be unfamiliar. Thus, before proceeding with our discussion of network models, we introduce the language used to describe networks and the measures (metrics) used to quantify their properties. We also illustrate several of the basic concepts in Figure 6.4. The definitions below are derived from Roberts (1976) and Newman (2003d). Wasserman and Faust (1994) also provide an extensive introduction to the language and techniques of network analysis.

6.3.1   Basic terms and structural components of networks

In Section 2.4.5.5 and Figure 2.5 we briefly introduced some of the most basic network terminology. Recall that when edges are used simply to indicate the presence of a link between two individuals (or nodes) the graph is said to be *undirected*. If, on the other hand, a link implies a connection in a specific direction, say A to B, B to A, or both, then the graph is called a *directed* graph. If, as suggested in Figure 2.5, weights are used to represent the strength of a particular connection, then the graph is called a *weighted* graph.

One question of interest in the study of social networks is whether it is possible to get from node (or individual) A to node B by following different edges of the network. In real social networks this corresponds to the chance that a piece of information or a pathogen can spread either directly or indirectly from one particular individual to another particular individual. The trail followed in going from A to B is called a *path*. If no node in the path is visited more than once, the path is called a *simple path*; one that ends at its starting point is called a *closed path*. A simple closed path, which begins and ends at the same point and never visits a particular node more than once, is also referred to as a *cycle*. The *path length* is defined to be the number of edges in a path. Figure 6.4 illustrates these concepts and several of those described in the following paragraphs.

Two nodes are *adjacent* to each other if they share an edge. Adjacent nodes have the potential to transmit information or pathogens directly between them. Node A is said to be *reachable* from node B if there is a path from B to A (this is sometimes called *pairwise connectedness*). In addition, all nodes that can be reached from a particular node are said to form a *component* of the graph. In a directed graph each node would have both an in-component (the set of other nodes from which the node can be reached) and an out-component (the set of other nodes that can be reached from the node in question).

Network analysts also have devised several measures of distance. For example, the simple distance, also known as the *geodesic distance*, is the length of the shortest path between two particular nodes, while the *diameter* of a graph is the length of the longest geodesic distance between any two nodes of the graph. The geodesic distance gives an idea about how long it might take for a particular person to become exposed to a pathogen transmitted by another person in the group;

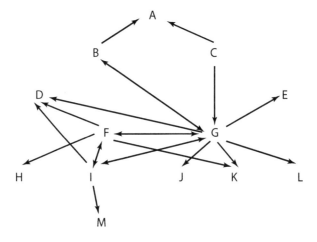

Simple path   C - G - L
Closed path   F - G - I - F (also a simple closed path)
Path length from G to M is 2 via node I or 3 via node F
The geodesic distance from G to M is 2

Node	Degree	In-degree	Out-degree	
A	2	2	0	
B	2	1	2	
C	2	0	2	
D	3	3	0	
E	1	1	0	
F	5	2	5	central node
G	9	4	8	central node
H	1	1	0	
I	4	2	4	central node
J	1	1	0	
K	2	2	0	
L	1	1	0	
M	1	1	0	

Figure 6.4 Examples of some of the basic network concepts described in the text.
The network here is the friendship network shown in Figure 6.3a.

the diameter relates more to group-level transmission potentials and determines in some sense how long chains of infection must be in order to span the population. One can also talk about the average geodesic distance of the network, which, in the disease context, describes the average distance between any two nodes. Similarly, the average diameter of the graph would say something about how long the longest chain of infection between all infected individuals to any susceptible individuals might be on average.

A particular node can have any number of edges connected to it up to one less than the total population size; the term *degree* is used to indicate the number of connected edges. If a graph is a directed graph, then it is possible to talk about both the in-degree and the out-degree for each node. Nodes with a high degree, especially in relation to other nodes, are said to be *central*; the corresponding term *centrality* (or more specifically, *degree centrality*) expresses which particular nodes are best connected to others. The latter term is often used to distinguish this simple measure of centrality from the many other measures of centrality that have been derived. In studies of social interactions, nodes with a central position in the network often have a higher degree of influence on network mediated processes (like the spread of diseases or information) than nodes that are less central.

The three concepts — adjacency, reachability (pairwise connectedness), and distance — are used frequently in mathematical analyses of network structures, and so they are commonly represented in matrix form. The elements of these matrices represent the relevant measure between the two nodes given by the row and column number of the element. For example, consider the network represented in Figure 6.4. Row 2, column 4 of the adjacency matrix indicates whether the nodes B and D are adjacent to one another (assuming each node is arrayed alphabetically along the rows and columns of the matrix). This element would equal 0 since there is no edge connecting the two nodes. The same row and column of the reachability matrix indicates whether B can be reached from D. This would also equal zero since it is not possible to go from D to any other node. On the other hand, it is possible to reach D from B by taking the path B - G - D, and so the element in row 4, column 2 of the reachability matrix would have the value 1. The element in row 4, column 2 of the distance matrix gives the distance between nodes D and B (however that distance is defined for the purpose of the study). An interesting feature of the adjacency matrix is that the powers of that matrix, i.e., A^t, give the number of paths of length t between the corresponding nodes.

6.3.2 Network metrics

The structural components described up to this point apply to one or a small number of nodes within the network. Network analysts have also derived a number of measures to characterize the overall structure of a network. One could argue that the graph diameter discussed above falls into this group because it takes into account the distance between all pairs of nodes, but most of the metrics described here are even more generalized.

Two nodes are connected if there is a path between them, and this concept extended to the entire network is its *connectedness*. Connectedness is one of the most fundamental properties of a network. Complete connectedness occurs if a path exists between every pair of nodes in the network. Furthermore, if for every pair of nodes, A and B, A can be reached from B and B can be reached from A, the network is said to possess strong connectedness. Other weaker degrees of connectedness are also possible. If one or more pairs of nodes in the network do not have a path between them, then the network is said to be disconnected.

Recall that the phrase "degree of a node" (or sometimes "connectivity of a node") is used to refer to the number of other nodes connected by an edge to a particular node. Let k_x designate the number of neighbors (connected nodes) of a given node, where x denotes the node of interest. Let p_k be the proportion of nodes in the network as a whole that have $k = 0, 1, 2, \ldots$ neighbors. The distribution of the p_k values describes the *connectivity* or *degree distribution* of the entire network. For example, the degree distribution of the network given in Figure 6.4 is determined as follows: There are 13 nodes in the network. As shown in Figure 6.4, none of those nodes have degree 0, 5 have degree 1, 4 have degree 2, 1 has degree 3, 1 has degree 4, 1 has degree 5, and 1 has degree 9. So the degree distribution is $[p_0, p_1, p_2, \ldots, p_9] = [0, \frac{5}{13}, \frac{4}{13}, \frac{1}{13}, \frac{1}{13}, \frac{1}{13}, 0, 0, 0, \frac{1}{13}]$.

If the degree distribution is broad, the network exhibits marked variation among the connectivities of different sites; in other words, some nodes possess only a few neighbors while others possess a lot. Such networks are often simply termed heterogeneous networks, although this term is not ideal since variation in the degree of nodes is not the only type of heterogeneity that a network can exhibit. For instance, in epidemiological studies there may be spatial heterogeneity in the network or heterogeneity in susceptibility and/or infectiousness across nodes. The degree distribution is often summarized in terms of its mean and variance. The average number of neighbors is sometimes written as $\langle k \rangle$ and the variance of the degree distribution as $\text{Var}(k)$.

One characteristic of networks that is of particular interest in studies of infectious disease transmission is the property of network transitivity or clustering. Transitivity refers to the fact that if two nodes are both connected to a third node, they are also likely to be connected to each other, thus forming a triangle (A is connected to B, B is connected to C, and C is connected to A). A similar concept is that of a triple, which arises whenever three nodes, A, B, and C, are connected to form a path of length three. All triangles are triples, but not all triples are triangles. Nodes F, G, and I in Figure 6.4 form a triangle; F, I, and M form a triple that is not a triangle. This phenomenon of transitivity can be colloquially expressed as "if you are my friend, your friends are likely to also be my friends" (and vice versa) (Feld, 1991; Newman, 2003a). Groups of nodes resulting from transitivity are often called *cliques*, although cliques need not always be of size three. For instance, a four-membered clique arises when two neighbors of two connected individuals are themselves connected, giving rise to a loop of length four in the network. In the context of infectious disease transmission, this concept captures the degree to which the occurrence of shared neighbors reduces the potential for secondary infections.

Network analysts have derived several metrics to measure the degree of clustering. For example, one such measure calculates a quantity ϕ, defined as the fraction of triples in the network that form triangles. Watts and Strogatz (1998) devised a similar measure that calculates a clustering coefficient for a particular node A by dividing the number of triangles connected to that node by the number of triples centered on that node. The network-wide clustering coefficient is then the simple average of all the individual clustering coefficients. This metric tends to weight the contributions of low-degree nodes more heavily than the quantity ϕ and can result in a measure that differs from ϕ quite significantly (Newman, 2003d).

Another network concept of importance for the study of infectious disease transmission is the concept of network resilience (Albert et al., 2000). This concept considers the impact of removing nodes from a network. Such removals can increase the typical length of paths, particularly if a highly central node is removed, and if enough nodes are removed the network can become fragmented into disconnected subcomponents. Such a concept can work to the advantage of disease control efforts by providing a way to identify individuals with the greatest potential to disrupt transmission chains. Those individuals can then be targeted for treatment or preventive actions.

In Sections 2.4.5 and 4.3.2.1 we discussed the kinds of mixing patterns that can occur within and between populations. Similar kinds of formulations arise when considering the connections among individuals or nodes within a network. As in our earlier discussion of mixing patterns, network mixing can be assortative (individuals/nodes are more likely to be connected to similar individuals/nodes), disassortative (individuals/nodes are more likely to be connected to dissimilar individuals/nodes), or random (there is no preference in connections among the nodes). The mixing pattern might be described in terms of spatial structure and the locations of individuals, in which case one might distinguish between local (assortative) and global (random) mixing. More generally, mixing can be described in terms of some other attribute of the population (Newman, 2002a).

Often models assume that the degree of individual nodes specifies the node type, and in such a case the mixing patterns are described in terms of how nodes of a particular degree are connected to nodes of other degrees. Such patterns are analogous to the activity level based mixing of the multigroup example described in Section 2.4.5, and they are most commonly discussed for networks with heterogeneous degree distributions.

Newman (2002b, 2003b) studied the properties of assortative mixing on networks both analytically and numerically. The following discussion is derived from some of this work. Consider a network with N nodes and degree distribution $p_0, p_1, p_2, \ldots$, where each p_k gives the proportion of nodes of degree k. The values of k are analogous to the activity levels, a_k, in the example in Section 2.4.5. The number of nodes that have degree k is equal to Np_k and each of these nodes contribute k connections to the total pool of available connections made by all nodes in the network. Thus, these individuals/nodes contribute kNp_k connections to the connection pool. The total number of available connections is $\sum_{k=0}^{\infty} kNp_k$. Since each interaction (represented by an edge in the graph) involves two nodes, this quantity is equal to twice the number of edges in the network. (Notice that there was an analogous factor of two that arose in the activity level based multigroup model discussed earlier.) The fraction of available connections that are made by nodes of degree k is given by

$$
\begin{aligned}
q_k &= \frac{kNp_k}{\sum_{j=0}^{\infty} jNp_j} \\
&= \frac{kp_k}{\sum_{j=0}^{\infty} jp_j} .
\end{aligned}
\tag{6.1}
$$

These quantities are analogous to the fractional activity levels described in our earlier example.

We previously defined proportionate mixing to be a mixing pattern where individuals have no preference for those with whom they interact. In the context of networks this means that the probability that a given connection of a node (or individual) is with another node of degree k is equal to q_k. As in the multigroup formulation, proportionate mixing within a network is sometimes called random mixing, but it should be realized that connections are chosen at random from the pool of available connections, i.e., from the population of connections, rather than by choosing individuals or nodes at random from the population. Since more highly connected nodes have more available connections than poorly connected nodes, they will be represented more often in the population of connections and will thus be "chosen" more often.

The set of all q_k describes the distribution of connectivities of nodes found by choosing edges at random from the network. Another way of saying this is that the q_k's describe the distribution of connectivities of nodes that are found by randomly choosing neighbors of randomly chosen nodes.

An interesting observation is that these randomly chosen neighbors have higher degree than randomly chosen members of the population. The average of the q_k can be calculated:

$$
\begin{aligned}
\sum_{k=0}^{\infty} k q_k &= \sum_{k=0}^{\infty} k \frac{k p_k}{\sum_{j=0}^{\infty} j p_j} \\
&= \frac{\sum_{k=0}^{\infty} k^2 p_k}{\sum_{j=0}^{\infty} j p_j} \\
&= \frac{\mathrm{Var}(k) + \langle k \rangle^2}{\langle k \rangle} \\
&= \langle k \rangle \left(1 + \mathrm{CV}_k^2 \right).
\end{aligned}
\tag{6.2}
$$

Here, CV_k denotes the coefficient of variation of the degree distribution.

The similarity between this result and the expression for R_0 that results from proportionate mixing in the multigroup model (Equation 2.20) should be noted. This result has long been known in the social network arena, where it has been expressed as "your friends have more friends than you do." This phenomenon is a consequence of the fact that, as discussed above, highly connected individuals are overrepresented in this pool and so a randomly chosen connection is more likely to be made to a highly connected individual than to one who is poorly connected.

Assortative and disassortative mixing can be defined relative to the q_k's of proportionate mixing. For these nonrandom mixing patterns, the probability that a given connection of an individual is with a person of degree k depends on the degree, k', of the first individual. We may write this probability as $q(k, k')$. For assortative mixing, the probability of a connection between two individuals of the same degree, $q(k, k)$, is greater than the connectivity of that degree alone, q_k, while the remaining $q(k, k')$ (connections between individuals of different degrees) are smaller than the corresponding q_k. For disassortative mixing, $q(k, k)$ is smaller than q_k.

6.4 MAJOR CLASSES OF NETWORKS

Although a number of epidemic models have incorporated actual networks derived from data of various sorts, most of the important general results about the impact of network structures on patterns of spread of infectious diseases across time and space have been derived from studies using theoretically based, ideal types of networks. In this section we provide an introduction to the most important of these networks, which are best seen as simple canonical models rather than realistic depictions of real-world networks. They provide a theoretical foundation for network studies that allows better understanding of the results derived from models using empirical data.

Perhaps the best known of these canonical network types are the small-world networks, which formalize the idea of "six degrees of separation" — the number of links between any two people in the world is likely to be no more than six. The idea has stimulated a Broadway play, *Six Degrees of Separation* (which was later adapted into a movie), popular games such as "Six Degrees of Kevin Bacon," or, for the mathematically inclined, the determination of the "Erdös number." In "Six Degrees of Kevin Bacon" the goal is to try to get to Kevin Bacon in no less than 6 links through the following strategy: pick an actor and a movie that actor has been in, then choose someone else in that movie and another movie they have been in, pick a third actor who appears in the second actor's other movie, etc. until a link is made to a movie in which Kevin Bacon appears. A person's "Erdös number" is determined by following a chain of collaborators on mathematical publications until Paul Erdös is reached. (Erdös was a highly prolific and eccentric mathematician who made major contributions to graph theory and other areas of mathematics. More on the "Erdös number" game can be found at the Erdös Number Project website, http://www.oakland.edu/enp/.)

Small-world networks are a relatively recent addition to the arsenal of canonical networks, however, and will be discussed in more detail below. We first describe two older and more general types of networks that are commonly used in epidemiological studies — random graphs and lattice models. Small-world networks form the third category we consider, and we follow this with a description of the newest network type to be brought into epidemic modeling, scale-free networks, as well as a few additional approaches.

6.4.1 Random graphs

Random graphs have received much attention in the mathematical graph theory literature, and much is known about their properties. Most of the concepts discussed in previous sections are derived from the analysis of such networks. A common kind of random graph, called the Erdös-Rényi random graph, is formed by randomly and independently connecting pairs of nodes within a population of N nodes (see Figure 6.5). The probability of any given pair of nodes being connected is represented by p. The number of neighbors of a given node is binomially distributed, with mean $(N - 1)p$. When N is large, the mean number of neighbors is well approximated by Np. Because connections between nodes are made randomly and without regard to the spatial location of nodes, random networks do not possess any real spatial structure. The population of nodes can be thought of as "well-mixed" in some sense, but it is important to realize that this does not mean that every node is connected to every other node.

The connectedness of an entire random graph is strongly influenced by the magnitude of the connection probability, p. When p is small, the random graph tends to consist of a set of disconnected components, but when p is large, most of the sites of the graph are connected in one giant component, although there may also be a few isolated small components and nodes. More formally, for large N, the random graph has a single giant component if and only if Φ is greater than one, where $\Phi = Np$ (Bollobás, 1985). This giant component then contains a proportion z of the population, where z is the largest root of

$$z = 1 - \exp(-\Phi z). \qquad (6.3)$$

This behavior is reminiscent of the transition that occurs at the $R_0 = 1$

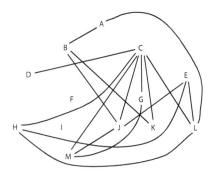

Figure 6.5 An example of a random graph linking the girls of Figure 6.3a. The graph was formed by assuming a probability of 0.2 for each possible link.

threshold in simple epidemic models. This correspondence between the construction of the random graph and the epidemic behavior of the Reed-Frost model is discussed in detail by Barbour and Mollison (1990).

While the diameter of a random graph has not been completely characterized under general conditions, both it and the average minimum path length (the average geodesic distance) appear to scale as $\log N/\log(Np)$ (Chung and Lu, 2001, 2002). This means that these parameters increase relatively slowly with increases in the number of nodes, which reflects the fact that connections between nodes are made independently of the distance between nodes. In addition to these features of random graphs, analyses have shown that cliques occur only rarely and the degree distribution has a relatively small variance (meaning that most nodes have a similar number of neighbors).

6.4.2 Lattice network models

A lattice is an arrangement of points or objects in a regular and periodic pattern in space. Usually lattices are represented as lines or as square or cubic grids (see Figure 6.6). In one dimension, individuals are regularly arranged on a line segment, with connections to their nearest neighbors on either side. A common model in population genetics, the stepping stone model, is an example of a one-dimensional lattice. In two dimensions, rectangular arrays are often employed, with the nodes of the graph usually occurring at the corners of the individual squares in the array. In many theoretical versions of two-dimensional lattice models, connections are assumed to occur between a particular node and its four (up, down, left, and right) or eight nearest neighbors (up, down, left, right, and diagonal neighbors). These two neighborhoods are known as the von Neumann and Moore neighborhoods, respectively (see Figure 6.6). Larger neighborhoods with connections made further away than nearest neighbors can also be defined, and other two-dimensional arrays, such as triangular or hexagonal lattices, can be employed. In addition, some representations of two-dimensional lattice models, commonly called cellular automata, place the nodes within the squares of the grid and do not explicitly show the edges linking nodes. Furthermore, in lattice models incorporating empirical data on nodal interactions, edges may appear only if there is an actual connection between the nodes involved.

If lattices are finite in size, then edge effects may become a problem because nodes on the edges of the lattice have fewer neighbors than nodes in the interior. Edge effects are sometimes avoided by the imposition of periodic boundary conditions. In the one-dimensional case, this corresponds to wrapping the line segment into a circle, making the first and last points neighbors. Analogous strategies are used for higher-dimensional lattices.

Connections within a lattice model are purely local in nature. Thus, paths between two nodes chosen at random tend to be long, with a large number of steps through intervening nodes. In other words, the average minimum path length is relatively long. In a one-dimensional lattice, this length is proportional to the population size. All interior nodes in a two-dimensional theoretical lattice (i.e., one that has the idealized, complete rectangular structure) have the same number of neighbors and thus possess the same degree, so the degree (or connectivity) distribution is nearly homogeneous (or completely homogeneous if edge effects are accounted for in some way). The same holds true for higher-dimensional lattices. The structure of regular lattice models is such that they tend to exhibit a fair degree of clustering or cliquishness. It is important to note, however, that the two-dimensional lattice with von Neumann neighborhoods exhibits cliquish behavior in the absence of triangles, indicating limitations in the common definition of a clique as a triangular group of connected nodes.

The simplest lattice network model describes a perfectly homogeneous environment, but, as in all kinds of graphs, different interaction strengths can be assigned to the connections. In one particularly interesting limiting case, which can be seen as a somewhat randomized version of the regular lattice, each of the possible connections allowed by the underlying lattice structure is actually made with probability p. This is the basis of the bond percolation model (Broadbent and Hammersley, 1957), which is a prominent technique for the mathematical analysis of lattice models.

As a lattice provides a particularly simple spatial geometry, modelers often employ this structure in simulation studies. It is important to note that many of these lattice models do not fall within the individual-based framework of this chapter. For instance, spatially continuous models are often discretized according to a rectangular lattice for the purposes of simulation. This discretized model is really a metapopulation model, with each cell representing a collection of individuals who are assumed to interact in a well-mixed fashion, but whose states need not be identical. (Notice that this differs from the situation in which the "individual" is a family: in such models, it is assumed that the different family members have the same disease statuses.)

6.4.3 Small-world networks

In the mid-1960s, Stanley Milgram, a psychologist at Yale University, began a series of experiments (Milgram, 1967; Travers and Milgram, 1969) that became the origin of the concept of "six degrees of separation" (although he did not use this phrase himself). The goal of these experiments was to see what length of a chain of persons would be required in order to send some documents from a participant in the study to some randomly assigned target individual. Milgram asked participants to pass the documents to someone they knew well, who would then pass them on to someone that they knew, etc. until the documents reached the target. Most of the packets were lost, but about one-fourth of them reached the target, passing through the hands of, on average, about 6 people. This work was one of the first demonstrations of what has now become widely known as the "small-world effect" (Newman, 2003d).

Milgram was not the first to propose the idea of the small-world effect, however. One of the earliest expressions of this idea occurred in a short story written by a Hungarian author, Frigyes Karinthy (1929), who challenged readers to find someone who could not be connected to him by a chain of five or fewer people (Barabási, 2003). In addition, according to Newman (2003d), Pool and Kochen (1978) developed the concept mathematically, and, although their work was published after Milgram conducted his experiments, preprints of the work had been

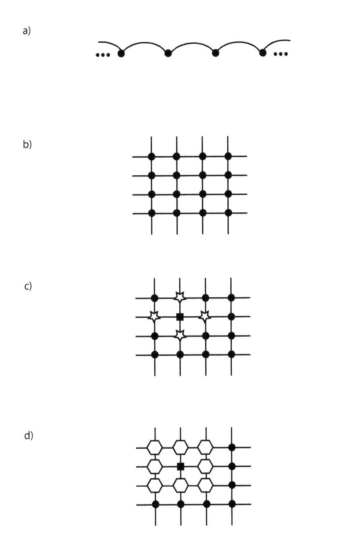

Figure 6.6 Examples of lattices and 2-dimensional lattice neighborhoods. a) 1-dimensional nearest-neighbor (or stepping stone) lattice model. b) 2-dimensional lattice. c) Von Neumann neighborhood surrounding the black square. d) Moore neighborhood surrounding the black square.

in circulation for a decade before Milgram's experiments were begun.

The small-world effect was first built into a network model by Watts and Strogatz (1998). This seminal paper has stimulated a large body of work on complex networks of all types, including epidemiological networks. Small-world models are intermediate in form between the random graph, representing the extreme of nonlocalized spatial structure and the regular lattice, which represents the extreme localized spatial structure. In the small-world network model most connections are local in nature, but there are also a (usually small) number of long-range connections.

One way to generate small-world networks is to start with a regular lattice and then either add new connections between random nodes of the lattice or rewire a small number of existing links by disconnecting them from their end node and relinking them to another randomly selected node. The Watts and Strogatz model considers an N-node one-dimensional lattice with periodic boundary conditions (in other words, the nodes are arranged on a circle). Each node is connected to those nodes that are within k places of it, so each node has $2k$ neighbors. Watts and Strogatz used the node rewiring mechanism to make the small-world network, with the constraint that the new end node of a rewired link could not be either the originating node or any nodes with which that node was already connected. The process of rewiring occurred by going through each edge in the graph successively and then determining, with probability θ, whether that edge would be rewired. On average the network resulting from such a process has $\theta k N$ new links; these new links are called shortcuts or "long range links" (Figure 6.7).

When θ equals zero, i.e., when no edges are broken and rewired, the network is simply a regular lattice. As discussed in the previous sections, in this case connections are entirely local, the path lengths are long, and the network exhibits a high degree of cliquishness. As θ approaches one, the network becomes a random network, and in this case it is well-mixed with short path lengths and low cliquishness.

The surprising finding of Watts and Strogatz's studies is that only a relatively small number of long-range connections are needed to reduce the average minimum path length of a lattice model to that of the corresponding random graph — a small number of nonlocal connections rapidly gives the otherwise locally connected lattice the global connectivity pattern typical of a random graph. In a one-dimensional situation, the diameter of the small-world network is seen to scale more like $\log N$, as seen in the random graph, than the linear scaling, N, of the lattice model. Since most connections are still local

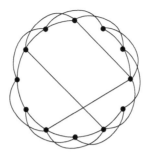

Figure 6.7 A small-world network. The base structure is a 12-node one-dimensional circular lattice with connections to the nearest 2 neighbors. Three of the edges of this base structure were disconnected and randomly rewired to a new node.

in nature, however, small-world networks tend to be cliquish.

In common with the random graph and lattice models, the degree distribution of the small-world network model is fairly peaked around its mean. In other words, few individuals have many more, or many fewer, neighbors than the mean.

Other algorithms have been developed for generating small-world networks. The simplest of these follows the same strategy as that used by Watts and Strogatz (1998), except that new edges are added rather than simply rewiring existing edges. In many cases this change makes little difference in the basic behavior of the model, but it does facilitate mathematical analysis of the network and its dynamics.

6.4.4 Scale-free networks

The three network types just discussed exhibit little or no heterogeneity with regard to the connectivity of individuals. Many real-world networks are quite unlike this, showing substantial variations in connectedness — while most individuals are poorly connected, a small number of individuals exhibit high connectivity (Barabási and Albert, 1999). One example of such a situation arises in sexual partnership networks, where the distributions of numbers of partnerships have long tails, with a few individuals (such as sex workers) having many more partners than the average (Liljeros et al., 2001; May and Anderson, 1988; Schneeberger et al., 2004).

Barabási and Albert (1999) devised a new network model, the scale-free network, that could be used to describe such heterogeneous situations. Their network is generated via a dynamic process that involves

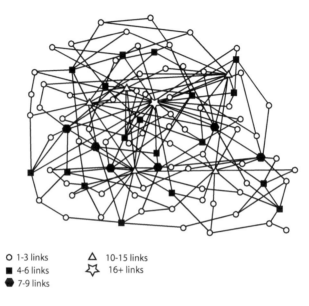

Figure 6.8 Example of a scale-free network. Redrawn from Lloyd and May (2001).

preferential attachment of nodes. New nodes are added to the network one at a time, and when they are introduced links are made to existing nodes, but with a preference for attachment to already well-connected nodes. This "rich get richer" process leads to a highly heterogeneous network in which most nodes have few neighbors, but a few have many neighbors (Figure 6.8). The degree distribution is (asymptotically) described by a power law of the form $p_k = Ak^{-3}$. The variance of this distribution is very large, becoming infinite as the number of individuals tends to infinity. Path lengths tend to be short in this network, mixing is global in nature rather than localized as in the lattice model, and the model tends to exhibit low levels of cliquishness.[1]

---

[1]It is important to note that although the observed distribution of numbers of sexual partnerships is highly skewed, there is disagreement about whether it can be represented as a scale free network (see Jones and Handcock (2003) and Liljeros et al. (2003)).

6.4.5 Other network types

Mixing patterns of real populations are usually much more complicated than those just described, exhibiting, for instance, nonrandom
mixing or hierarchical structure. Although less attention has been
directed towards such situations, network structures have been described that address these complications. For instance, Ball et al.
(1997) describe a population with two levels of mixing, local and
global. Individuals are most likely to interact with (and, hence, infect or acquire infection from) individuals in some local neighborhood.
There is a smaller chance that they interact with any other individual
in the population. Different descriptions of the local neighborhood
are employed: in one, it is assumed that the population is made up
of a collection of n discrete groups, and another assumes that individuals are located on a circle, with their local neighborhood being
the two individuals to their left and right. Notice that the first formulation could be viewed as a metapopulation model, albeit one for
which within-patch structure is explicitly considered, and the second
provides an instance of the small-world model of Watts and Strogatz
(1998).

The scale-free network generated by Barabási and Albert (1999)
exhibits a random mixing pattern. Many variants of their process have
been suggested, giving rise to epidemiologically interesting network
types, including locally spatially structured networks exhibiting high
levels of heterogeneity (Rozenfeld et al., 2002; Warren et al., 2002)
and highly heterogeneous networks that exhibit nonrandom mixing
patterns (Klemm and Eguiluz, 2002).

6.5 THE INFLUENCE OF NETWORKS ON THE DYNAMICS OF EPIDEMIC SPREAD

Network models are most commonly used within the context of sexually transmitted diseases, such as HIV/AIDS (for example, Kretzschmar and Morris, 1996; Morris and Kretzschmar, 1995, 1997), gonorrhea (Kretzschmar et al., 1996), or chlamydia (Kretzschmar et al.,
1996; Kretzschmar, 2002). It should be realized, however, that for
many of these models, the networks might only have a loose connection with the geographic structure of the population. In fact, applications of network models to the geographic spread of human infectious
diseases are relatively rare, an issue we will return to in the last section
of this chapter. Consequently, our discussion of the insights from net-

work models will mostly focus on more theoretical analyses, although we motivate that discussion with a brief look at STD models. Full discussion of STD models is beyond the scope of this book, however — both because their applications to geographic spread are limited and also because the important public health implications of AIDS and other STDs in today's society have resulted in a huge body of research. For more in-depth examples of some of the research being done in this area, interested readers are encouraged to consult Morris (2004b) or a special issue of the journal *Sexually Transmitted Diseases* (Volume 27, Issue 10, 2000) devoted to network models for STDs.

The structure of sexual partnership networks differs in several important ways from that of the networks used to describe the spread of other infectious diseases. For example, as mentioned previously, sexual networks possess a high level of heterogeneity because most individuals have only a small number of sexual partners over their lifetimes, but an appreciable number have many partners (see, for example, Liljeros et al., 2001). The highly sexually active individuals are responsible for a disproportionate number of transmission events. Such individuals are likely to provide bridges between different communities (for example, IV drug users and the non-drug-using population), and they may also provide a mechanism by which the spatial spread of infection can be considerably enhanced.

In addition, sexual transmission must, of necessity, include constraints on the direction of potential transmission that are not necessarily present for diseases spread through other means. Obviously, if considering a purely heterosexual population, transmission can only occur from male to female and vice versa, but asymmetry in transmission occurs for more subtle reasons as well. In real populations sexual behavior occurs homosexually as well as heterosexually, but the frequency of such behaviors varies markedly and so the frequency of transmission from male-to-male and female-to-female will be much lower than male-to-female or female-to-male. In addition, it has been reported that the transmission process between sexes is often asymmetric. As an example, the risk of transmission of HIV from males to females is thought to be higher than in the reverse direction (Peterman et al., 1988), although at least some studies suggest that this is not always the case (see, for example, Gray et al., 2001).

Another complication that must be dealt with in network models for sexually transmitted diseases is that individuals who are involved in long-term monogamous relationships are, for the most part, removed from the large-scale disease transmission process. If both partners are fully monogamous and susceptible then there is no way for either to become infected, and even if one partner became infected during or before the onset of the partnership, as long as both partners remain monogamous, transmission could occur only to the uninfected partner and no further. Because of this, long-term monogamous relationships result in a large number of pairs disconnected from others in the sexual partnership network.

The earliest attempts to model sexual networks involved the use of what are called pair formation models. These kinds of models have been part of the arsenal in demographic studies of marriage and fertility for some time, but they were first introduced into epidemiological studies by Dietz and Hadeler (1988). In the model of Dietz and Hadeler, the population is divided into single males and females of different disease statuses and male-female pairs. The model also keeps track of the disease status of both members of a pair. As in other population-based models, individuals within a group are not explicitly considered; thus, the Dietz-Hadeler model is essentially a multigroup population-based model with a specific implied underlying network consisting of isolated nodes (single individuals) and pairs of nodes joined by edges (the sexual pairs). In addition, consistent with other population-based models, variation among individuals within each group is ignored. Contrary to many population-based models, however, the population is not well-mixed for the purposes of disease transmission; single individuals are not at risk of exposure and individuals in pairs are only at risk from the other member of their pair and do not become exposed to infectious individuals outside their pair at a particular time (although they can dissolve a particular partnership and enter into another with someone who is infectious). In addition, the Dietz-Hadeler and similar models are generally based on the assumption that sexual partnerships are nonoverlapping, but in many human populations having multiple sexual partners (often referred to as concurrency) is a common occurrence or even the norm for some proportion of the population. The effect of concurrent relationships on disease spread has been of much interest in network studies of STD transmission (for example, Bauch and Rand, 2001; Chick et al., 2000; Kretzschmar and Morris, 1996) and some of the most interesting work in this area relates to this question.

Results from analysis of network models for STD transmission indicate that the factors that have the strongest influence on disease patterns are the average number of sexual partners, the concurrency of partnerships, the duration of partnerships, and the overall connectivity of a network (Doherty et al., 2006; Ghani and Garnett, 2000; Kretzschmar, 2000). Ghani and Garnett (2000) showed that network structure affected the risk of acquiring infection differently from the risk of transmission of infection. In particular, measures of local network structure, such as the centrality of an individual had a greater impact on the risks of acquiring infection, while more global measures of network structure, such as connectivity, had greater effects on the risk of transmitting infection.

Kretzschmar and colleagues showed that the degree of concurrency had significant effects on the rate of growth at the beginning of an epidemic, on the number of infected individuals at any time t, and on the number of nodes in the largest network component (Kretzschmar et al., 1994; Kretzschmar and Morris, 1996; Morris and Kretzschmar, 1995). Their results indicated that as the average level of concurrent partnerships increases, the time between successive partnerships and the duration of individual partnerships become less significant forces in determining patterns of epidemic spread; the greater availability of partners when the probability of concurrency is high decreases the chance that infection chains will be broken before transmission to new individuals occurs.

Simulation results of Doherty et al. (2006) showed that concurrency was most important for the lowest activity groups. In addition, the relationship between mixing patterns and concurrency was not a simple one — some mixing patterns exacerbated the effects of concurrency, others reduced those effects. Their conclusions were similar to those of Kretzschmar and colleagues — in general, sexual mixing facilitates the spread of sexually transmitted diseases through a population, while concurrency expedites transmission by shortening the time between successive transmissions from an infected individual to susceptibles, particularly during periods of high infectiousness.

6.6 THEORETICAL ANALYSIS OF NETWORK MODELS

As has been shown above, as long as a network is not too large and complex, it is easy to visualize its structures using a graph, but, in general, mathematical analyses of the effects of network structure on disease transmission patterns are not easy to perform. In fact, much of the study of network behavior has centered on simulation approaches. Many of these studies offer few general insights, and, in addition, it is almost always very difficult to determine the real-world network structure and appropriate transmission parameters. Nonetheless, as we describe in our applications chapters, individual-based simulations are being used increasingly to study the nature of infectious disease transmission in human populations. There remains an ongoing desire to gain more general understanding of the impact of network structure, however, and several approximation techniques have been developed to aid in this task. In this section we describe a few of the most important of these techniques.

6.6.1   Mean field approaches

The approximation techniques used in theoretical analyses of network structures necessarily involve considerably simplified descriptions of the network. For example, it might be assumed that cliques are rare or absent or that there are no loops in the network. A common strategy used in the analysis of epidemiological network models is to simplify a network by subdividing it into classes according to individuals' connectivities, which represent differing activity levels. The resulting model is exactly the heterogeneous population-level model described earlier, and so its properties (such as the importance of the mixing patterns between different activity classes and the impact of heterogeneity upon R_0) are quite familiar. In the statistical physics literature models such as this are known as "mean field" models. It is important to note that this approach disregards any local structure present in the network. In addition, in mean field analyses of STD models, all details of the timing of partnerships, and particularly whether they overlap, are disregarded by this population-level approach. Thus, this analysis technique cannot address the issue of concurrency, which, as we have discussed above, has important implications for the spread of sexually transmitted diseases.

6.6.2   Pair approximation methods

In recent years new mathematical techniques have been devised that allow more direct analyses of network models. One such technique is the moment closure approximation (see, for example, Bauch and Rand, 2001; Bauch, 2002, 2005; Ellner et al., 1998b; Keeling, 1999b; Matsuda et al., 1992; Rand, 1999; Sato et al., 1994). The first step in this technique is to write down equations that describe how the numbers of susceptible and infectious individuals change on a network of neighboring pairs of individuals. The model represented by these equations does not simply model the numbers of susceptible and infectious individuals; rather, it tracks the number of susceptible/susceptible, susceptible/infectious, and infectious/infectious pairs.[2]

The equations of the pair approximation model that describe how the overall numbers of susceptible and infectious individuals change include terms involving the numbers of each type of pair (S-S, S-I, I-R, etc.). This is hardly surprising since the spread of a disease on a network depends on the configuration of pairs of individuals, with transmission requiring a susceptible individual to be adjacent to an infectious individual. In a similar way, the equations describing how the number of pairs changes over time depend on the configuration of triples (e.g., the number of susceptible/infectious/susceptible triples), and equations describing changes in triples depend on the configuration of quadruples.

Theoretically, this process leads to an infinite number of equations, so, in order to make it manageable, the process is truncated at some point. This truncation is called a closure approximation. Pair correlation equations are obtained by employing a pair approximation, which relates the numbers of triples to lower order quantities in an appropriate way for the network under consideration. Notice that correlation models are of much higher dimension than their mean field counterparts — while the standard SIR model in a population of constant size is described by two independent coupled ODEs, the corresponding pair approximation model contains five (Keeling, 1999b).

In certain cases, additional approximations can be made to pair correlation models that reduce the description of the local spatial structure to a single variable (Keeling et al., 1997; Keeling, 1999b). The models that result can be viewed as modifications of the mass action population-level model. Their simplicity facilitates analysis and offers insights into how the correlation structure develops over the course of an epidemic and how this alters the mass action description of transmission.

A pair approximation approach can also be employed when transmission dynamics operate on several spatial scales (called "multiscale pair models" by Ellner (2001)) and such an approach can be extended to cover situations in which there is marked heterogeneity in the network's degree distribution (Bauch, 2002; Eames and Keeling, 2002). In the latter case, the number of variables in the model increases considerably, although it is possible to simplify the situation somewhat to enable some analyses (Eames and Keeling, 2002).

Pair approximation methods have also been used in more detailed

---

[2]The Dietz-Hadeler model described above also used this type of formulation, although a moment closure approximation was not used to analyze its behavior.

studies of the effects of concurrency (Bauch and Rand, 2001), where they allow analytic exploration of epidemic properties. For instance, expressions for the final size of an epidemic in a concurrent network are provided, together with improved expressions for R_0 that account for network structure. In a further refinement, Bauch (2002) extended this analysis to consider heterogeneous networks (see also Eames and Keeling, 2002). Importantly, this model retained information on the configuration of triples (i.e., it employs a triple approximation), increasing the accuracy of the approximation and enabling the accuracy of the pair approximation to be assessed. Bauch found that, in several situations, the pair approximation is seriously deficient. He argued that in these situations the triple approximation must instead be used, and he issued a general warning regarding the need to include error estimates whenever approximations (such as the pair approximation) are made.

6.6.3 Percolation theory

Percolation theory, another common method used in the physical sciences, has provided many analytic insights into the behavior of individual-based models and, in particular, network models (Grimmett, 1999; Stauffer and Aharony, 1992). Percolation models were first formulated by Broadbent and Hammersley (1957) to address whether a liquid can permeate a porous stone, and much of the discussion of this approach is phrased in terms of this application. Such models are applicable, however, to a wide range of situations in which the flow of some quantity (e.g., information, electrical current, or fire) through a population of interacting individuals (e.g., a computer network, an electrical circuit, or a forest) is of interest.

The original model, bond percolation on the two-dimensional square lattice, considers percolation on some portion of a square lattice, where sites are connected to their four nearest neighbors. The model assumes that only some edges are broad enough for water to pass; edges are either "open" or "closed," with each edge having a probability p of being open. A given site, x, found in the interior of the lattice, is said to be wetted if there is a path from x to the exterior of the stone along open edges. Percolation theory is concerned with deriving conditions under which most, or all, of the lattice sites are wetted.

Although bond percolation on a square lattice has received the most attention in the literature, percolation models can be considerably more general. For instance, they can be described for more general network structures, such as random graphs. Indeed, an alternative construction of the random graph of Section 6.4.1 involves starting with a completely connected graph and allowing edges to be open with probability p. Percolation can also be described in terms of the properties of sites (in which case they are called site percolation models): given some lattice, sites can be open or closed to the passage of the substance with probability p. Further generalizations are possible. For example, mixed models allow both sites and edges to be open or closed, inhomogeneous models allow the probability p to vary across a lattice, and so on. Despite these additional complexities, many of these models behave in ways reminiscent of the simplest model.

In some instances, percolation models are directly analogous to individual-based descriptions of disease transmission. As discussed above, the Reed-Frost model can be mapped onto the random graph model (Barbour and Mollison, 1990), which can itself be viewed as a percolation model. Earlier results of Kuulasmaa (1982) and Grassberger (1983) established the correspondence between the spread of a fixed infectious period SIR-type infection on a given network and bond percolation on that network. The probability of an edge being open in the bond percolation problem corresponds to the probability that an infectious individual will, at some point over the course of infection, infect a susceptible individual to whom he or she is connected. The transmission probability has been called the transmissibility of the infection (Newman, 2002b), and is written as T. If transmission occurs at rate β along an edge and an individual is infectious for exactly τ time units, then the transmissibility, T, is equal to $1 - e^{-\beta\tau}$.

In the broader setting of a general infectious period distribution, the transmissibility of infection is given by

$$T = 1 - \int_0^\infty f(t)e^{-\beta t}\, dt\,. \tag{6.4}$$

Here, $f(t)$ is the probability density function describing the infectious period distribution. Kuulasmaa (1982) made the important observation that the bond percolation model does not apply in the general setting (see also Diekmann et al., 1998a). Use of a nonfixed infectious period distribution leads to dependence between transmission events from individuals to their susceptible neighbors. This nonindependence is nicely illustrated in an example given by Mollison and Kuulasmaa (1985). Consider an infectious period distribution that is highly variable, so that some individuals have a long infectious period and others have a short duration of infection. The limiting case of this distribution, which we dub "all-or-nothing," would have some

fraction, f, of the population having an extremely long infectious period, leading to all of their neighbors becoming infected. On the other
hand, the remaining $1 - f$ would recover before any of their neighbors
became infected. So, knowing whether or not transmission occurs to
one neighbor tells us whether transmission occurs to the rest of the
neighbors. This corresponds to the site percolation model. Kuulasmaa (1982) showed that the fixed duration of infection model and the
all-or-nothing model bracket the general infectious period model —
its behavior lies somewhere between the two.

A central result of percolation theory is the existence of threshold
behavior (also known as critical behavior in the physical literature).
For instance, in the simple bond percolation model, it can be shown
that there exists a critical value of p, written p_C, at which a qualitative
change in the system's behavior occurs (Broadbent and Hammersley,
1957; Hammersley, 1957, 1959). When p is below p_C, the lattice is
mainly made up of small, disconnected clusters of sites. As p increases
above p_C, the clusters merge into one connected open cluster (known
as the giant component of the lattice). This behavior is clearly reminiscent of, and is directly analogous to the $R_0 = 1$ threshold behavior
exhibited by simple epidemic models; it is also reminiscent of the
random graph's threshold behavior.

In the correspondence between bond percolation and the fixed duration of infection epidemic model, the occurrence of a giant component
corresponds to the potential for a major outbreak of infection to occur
(Andersson, 1997, 1998; Barbour and Mollison, 1990; Diekmann et al.,
1998a). Above threshold, the fraction of the network's sites that are
in the giant component is equal to the size of a major outbreak,[3] if it
occurs, and the chance that introduction of infection (to a randomly
chosen individual) will lead to a major outbreak. Below threshold,
the size distribution of clusters is equal to the distribution of sizes of
minor outbreaks. An important difference that arises for models with
nonfixed infectious periods is that the size of a major outbreak no
longer equals the probability of the occurrence of a major outbreak
(Diekmann et al., 1998a).

Local spatial structure of a network, such as short distance loops
(cliques), complicates calculation of percolation thresholds. Many
analyses assume the absence of such loops, in which case infection
(at least during its early stages) spreads across a network in a tree-

---

[3]It is common in epidemic models to use the fraction of a population affected
to represent the size of an outbreak. It is in that sense that we refer to outbreak
size here.

like fashion. This spread can be described using a branching process model (Diekmann et al., 1998a). As discussed in Chapter 2, generating functions underlie much of the theory of branching processes and so it should not be surprising that generating functions underlie the main analytic methods of percolation theory.

Percolation theory can also be used to address more general questions. The original bond percolation model contains no notion of the timescale on which spread occurs. It is phrased in terms of static properties of the system, and so can be used to address questions of whether disease spread is possible and, if so, the likely size of an epidemic. A natural extension of the model, as provided by the spatial contact model of Harris (1974), introduces a description of the time course of infection, and can be used to address dynamical questions such as the speed at which a disease propagates through a population.

6.7 THE BASIC REPRODUCTIVE NUMBER IN NETWORK MODELS

Expressions for the basic reproductive number can be derived for the different network types using the basic approaches we have discussed in this chapter. In general, the concept is most relevant for networks with a local tree structure (in which case local correlations are not an issue), but it has been applied to networks of a variety of types, albeit with suitable caveats.

The mean field approximation provides the simplest route to obtain estimates of the basic reproductive number for networks, although it can be inadequate in some cases (see, for example, Ball and Neal, 2008). Recall that the mean field approximation leads to a multi-group model and that the latter is formulated in terms of the rate at which an individual makes contacts. In the network context this rate is re-interpreted in terms of the degrees of individuals. In a homogeneous setting, in which each individual has k neighbors, the mean field approach gives the following expression for R_0:

$$R_0 = \frac{\beta}{\gamma} k \,.$$
(6.5)

In a heterogeneous network with random mixing, the mean field expression for R_0 is

$$R_0 = \frac{\beta}{\gamma} \langle k \rangle (1 + CV^2) \,.$$
(6.6)

Here $\langle k \rangle$ is the average number of neighbors of nodes within the network and CV is the coefficient of variation of the number of neighbors. This is very similar to the expression for R_0 derived from the proportionate mixing model in Section 2.5, which is not surprising since the mean field model is just a multigroup heterogeneous population model. As was the case for the latter model, Equation 6.6 shows that increasing heterogeneity in the network increases the value of R_0.

Considering the case of scale-free networks, recall that they exhibit a high degree of heterogeneity, with most nodes poorly connected, but a small number very highly connected. Because of this heterogeneity, the value of R_0 is considerably inflated compared to the value predicted when using just the average connectivity. In fact, as the number of nodes in a scale-free network increases, the variance of the degree distribution diverges and so R_0 becomes infinite (Lloyd and May, 2001; May and Lloyd, 2001; Pastor-Satorras and Vespignani, 2001a). This leads to the result that infections can always spread on a true scale-free network as long as the transmission parameter, β, is nonzero (Pastor-Satorras and Vespignani, 2001b). In other words, the $R_0 = 1$ threshold does not exist in a scale-free network of infinite size. When such a network is of finite size, the variance is finite but large. In this case the epidemic threshold does exist, but only at very small values of β. Eguiluz and Klemm (2002) showed also that local spatial structure and nonrandom mixing can lead to scale-free networks with threshold effects.

The mean field approximation, based on the multigroup model, does not properly account for the repeated nature of contacts — an individual with connectivity k has a fixed set of k neighbors and so R_0 can never be greater than $k-1$. The mean field approximation centers on the rate of making contacts, however, and so with this formulation R_0 can be arbitrarily large.

Moving beyond mean field approximations, lattice models were the model type of choice in the earliest attempts at using individual-based models to calculate epidemic thresholds and spatial wave speeds. This setting has generated considerable interest, partly reflecting the fact that these models provide the fundamental representation of disease transmission that continuous models, such as the reaction-diffusion model, attempt to approximate. Most of this work has concerned the contact model of Harris (1974), for which lattice sites are either occupied (infected) or unoccupied (susceptible). Occupied sites become unoccupied (i.e., recover) after an average of one time unit, while occupied sites can cause neighboring unoccupied sites to become occupied at rate λ.

For the one-dimensional contact process, it has been proven that there is a critical value of λ, written as λ_C, such that disease persistence and disease invasion following the introduction of a single infectious individual is only possible for $\lambda > \lambda_C$. In this case, a wave of disease spreads outwards, to the left and right of the point of initial introduction, at (asymptotic) velocity between $\lambda - \lambda_C$ and $\lambda - 1$. For this model, the quantity R_0 can be shown to be approximately equal to $2\lambda/(1 + \lambda)$, with λ_C approximately equal to 1.649.

The corresponding mean field model predicts that $\lambda_C = 0.5$. As might be expected, disease spread occurs more readily when the population is well mixed — disease transmission is hindered by local spatial structure. Improved approximations to λ_C can be obtained using pair approximation techniques (Matsuda et al., 1992) since these account for some aspects of local spatial structure. The pair approximation approach gives $\lambda_C = 1.0$. A further improvement can be obtained using a modified pair approximation technique, the pair-edge approximation (Ellner et al., 1998b), which gives $\lambda_C = 1.71$, which is in very good agreement with the true value of λ_C. Similarly, use of pair and pair-edge approximations provide better estimates of wave speeds than those provided by the deterministic mean field model.

For more general network types, analyses can be carried out to calculate R_0 using percolation theory or branching process theory. As mentioned above, these analyses typically assume that short loops are absent. Further, it is generally assumed that the network is randomly mixed (as discussed above, this means that connections are chosen randomly from within the pool of available connections, not by choosing individual nodes at random). Perhaps the simplest case is that of a randomly mixed network in which each individual has exactly k neighbors (Diekmann et al., 1998a), for which the basic reproductive number is given by

$$R_0 = T(k - 1). \qquad (6.7)$$

Here, T is the transmissibility of the infection, as defined in Section 6.6.3. Notice that, unlike the formula derived using the mean field approximation, the basic reproductive number is proportional to the number of neighbors minus one. This is because, except for the initial infectious individual, each infectious individual must have acquired infection from one of their neighbors, and they can have at most $k - 1$ susceptible neighbors.

Andersson (1997, 1998) showed that in a randomly mixed heterogeneous network, the basic reproductive number can be written as

$$R_0 = T\left(\frac{\langle k^2 \rangle}{\langle k \rangle} - 1\right). \tag{6.8}$$

As before, $\langle k \rangle$ denotes the average number of neighbors of nodes and $\langle k^2 \rangle$ denotes the average of the squares of those numbers of neighbors. Using the result that $\text{Var}(k) = \langle k^2 \rangle - \langle k \rangle^2$, the expression for the basic reproductive number can be written as

$$R_0 = T(\langle k \rangle(1 + \text{CV}^2) - 1). \tag{6.9}$$

These results were later derived using percolation theory (Newman, 2002b, 2003d), together with expressions for the final sizes of epidemics on these networks.

6.8 INFECTION CONTROL ON NETWORKS

The basic structure of networks has definite implications for the spread and control of infectious diseases spreading across those networks. Intuitively, it should be clear that if the average distance between individuals is short, then a disease will spread faster than in networks with a longer average distance; in the latter case, the disease must spread through a greater number of intermediate individuals in order to traverse the population.

Analyses of epidemic spread across different kinds of networks has confirmed this intuition. In particular, infections spread much more quickly on random graphs than on lattices. They spread quickly on small-world networks as well, especially in comparison to lattice models, since the addition of the long-range links in those networks dramatically shortens the average distance between nodes (Figure 6.9).

The frequency of cliques on a network also affects the speed of spread of an infection. As discussed earlier, in cliques (or clusters) small sets of nodes will be tightly connected to each other, but less so to other such groups and to other individual nodes. In such a case, a disease has the potential to spread rapidly through the clique, but the infectious individuals within a clique will quickly find a diminishing supply of susceptibles to whom they can pass the infection. This dramatically reduces the population-level potential for secondary infections.

Such a result was seen by Sattenspiel (1987a,b) in her study of the spread of day care hepatitis in Albuquerque, New Mexico. Both

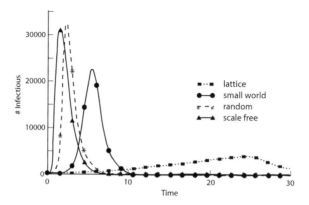

Figure 6.9 Epidemic curves resulting from disease spread on a random graph, a regular lattice, a small-world network, and a scale-free network. The transmission rate, β, and the recovery rate, γ, were the same for all models, and the average number of neighbors was fixed at 8. The small-world network involved a rewiring of 1% of the nodes.

mathematical analyses and simulation results showed that when most children attending a day care center lived only a short distance from the center (i.e., the center was highly localized), those children were at greater risk for becoming infected once the virus entered the day care center population than were children who attended centers drawing from a wider geographic range. The high risk of children attending localized centers was due to the fact that these children represented a highly clustered social group that maintained its structure not only in the day care center, but also in the home neighborhood, which was in the vicinity of the day care center.

Heterogeneity in the degree or number of neighbors of individuals also can enhance the spread of infection through the network. Highly connected nodes serve as foci for transmission, and when an individual with high degree becomes infected, a disease can spread rapidly to the rest of the network, even if most individuals in the network are poorly connected. If most individuals are poorly connected, however, then it may take some time for the epidemic to take off in the network, because of a lag in getting to the small number of highly connected individuals.

These general insights on the role of network structure on patterns of spread can be applied towards the task of assessing the potential effectiveness of different control strategies. For example, infections tend to spread locally on a lattice; thus, control measures that are directed at localized subgroups of the network are likely to be fairly effective. Unfortunately, analysis of small-world networks shows that only a few long-range contacts are needed in order to dramatically reduce the effectiveness of such localized control strategies. If the degree of different individuals in a network is highly variable (i.e., the network is highly heterogeneous), then, at the very minimum, effective control strategies must target the most highly connected individuals.

One of the most interesting network concepts that affects disease control strategies is the idea of network resilience. Recall from Section 6.3.2 that resilience refers to the ability of a network to withstand the removal of nodes. Vaccination, a common control strategy for infectious diseases, can be considered to be the removal of some number of nodes from a network, and vaccination targeted at those individuals at highest risk corresponds to removing nodes that possess high degree (Newman, 2003d). The impact of this was addressed by Pastor-Satorras and Vespignani (2002), who showed that networks tend to be highly vulnerable to removal of highly connected nodes (i.e., they are not resilient to such removals). Thus, vaccination targeted at these individuals is likely to be especially effective (thus validating theoretically a well-known and long-followed public health practice). The difficulty arises in determining who those highly connected nodes are and how to design a vaccination program that actually targets the intended individuals.

6.9   WHY AREN'T THERE MORE APPLICATIONS OF NETWORK MODELS FOR SPATIAL SPREAD?

It should be clear from this chapter that networks are an excellent way to model the patterns of interactions among individuals and how those patterns influence disease transmission within populations. So why are applications of network models to the geographic spread of infectious diseases, especially human infectious diseases, relatively uncommon in the epidemiological literature? In short, the major reasons for this are time and money. Determining the structure of social networks is very expensive, time-intensive, and complicated. Network studies require large amounts of detailed population data, and such data are not easily accessible or available. Remember that it is not only necessary to have information on every member of a population — information about every person's contacts and the circumstance of those contacts is also required.

Consider the Toronto SARS epidemic we discussed at the beginning of this chapter, for example. Varia et al. (2003) collected epidemiological data on 128 probable and suspected cases of the disease that were associated with a single hospital outbreak in Toronto. Forty-seven of these cases occurred in hospital staff. Imagine the number and variety of contacts each of those 47 cases would have (to say nothing about the remaining 81 cases). The ill staff members would have had numerous contacts within the hospital with both patients and other staff members, and they would also have had additional contacts within their households and with friends, acquaintances, fellow bus riders if that was how they got to work, etc. It is easy to see that even for a relatively small outbreak such as the 2003 SARS epidemic in Toronto, it would be a daunting task to determine fully the underlying contact network involved in disease spread. Clearly, efficient methods for estimating network structures are crucial in such situations. The variety of issues surrounding this problem are discussed in the many excellent papers found in Morris's book, *Network Epidemiology: A Handbook for Survey Design and Data Collection* (Morris, 2004a), and there are also substantive and insightful discussions related to this issue in Ghani and Garnett (1998) and Ghani et al. (1998).

In addition, placing the network structure in the context of geographic spread vastly increases the amount of data necessary to parameterize the model. In such a case, each geographic location being modeled would require detailed social network data. Most researchers do not have sufficient time, money, or computer power to incorporate a full network structure over any appreciable spatial dimension.

This does not mean that the task of developing network approaches for spatial models should be abandoned, however. Within the last decade it has become increasingly clear that network modeling efforts are a necessary supplement to more traditional approaches to modeling infectious disease transmission. More and better data sets are becoming available and new ways of approximating network and/or geographic structure are being devised, but there is still much work to be done. In fact, it could be argued that this is one of the most rapidly growing areas of epidemiological research today.

The detailed data needed for network models are more often available for diseases that affect farm animals. Given the economic significance of many veterinary infections, efficient mechanisms exist for rapid notification of disease and implementation of control measures. Information on the movement of farm animals (for instance, between farms and markets) is often collected in some detail and collated at a national level, particularly when government subsidies are provided to producers of food. As a consequence, veterinary infections often provide high-quality data sets for epidemiological analysis.

One of the best examples of the way that epidemiological data, including network data, have been used within a modeling framework is the 2001 U.K. outbreak of foot-and-mouth disease. This data set was sufficiently detailed to allow the deployment of several types of highly sophisticated models and statistical analyses, which were used not only to monitor the growing epidemic, but also to suggest and direct disease control policies at the national level (Ferguson et al., 2001a,b; Keeling et al., 2001). This epidemic, including a description of the epidemic itself, the official response to it (including modeling efforts), and the aftermath of that response, is the centerpiece of our next chapter.

Chapter Seven

Spatial Models and the Control of
Foot-and-Mouth Disease

In the middle of February 2001, the Official Veterinary Surgeon at a slaughterhouse in Essex, U.K., noticed that several recently slaughtered pigs were lame. This was a primary symptom suggestive of a particularly feared disease of domesticated animals, foot-and-mouth disease (FMD), that had not been reported in the country for 34 years. Suspicion was high enough that the slaughterhouse was immediately shut down and all remaining pigs were examined for the disease. Examination confirmed the presence of the disease and, although affected pigs originated from three different regions, most appeared to have been infected at the slaughterhouse itself. Further investigation traced the source of the epidemic to a pig-fattening unit in Northumberland that had sent 35 sows to the Essex slaughterhouse a few days before the disease was recognized. Direct spread of the disease to neighboring farms occurred by aerosol transmission or by transport on vehicles or personnel, with subsequent infections of both cattle and sheep (Gibbens et al., 2001).

Unfortunately, FMD produces very few lesions in infected sheep, and by the time it was recognized in the source and neighboring farms, infected sheep had been sent to six different markets in England, one in Wales, and several dealers' premises (Davies, 2002). Although a nationwide ban on movement of susceptible animals was instituted by the third week of February, it was not enough to prevent the development of a widespread epidemic that quickly spread throughout England and Wales and also reached Scotland, Northern Ireland, France, the Netherlands, the Republic of Ireland, and Germany (Davies, 2002; Gibbens et al., 2001) (Figure 7.1). The epidemic peaked in early April and largely subsided by the end of April, although it did not die out completely until the end of September (Davies, 2002) (Figure 7.2).

The 2001 epidemic devastated the U.K. livestock industry (Keeling et al., 2001). A similar epidemic occurred in the country in 1967, so authorities were well aware of the potential for foot-and-mouth disease to cause problems with wide-ranging and long-lasting economic

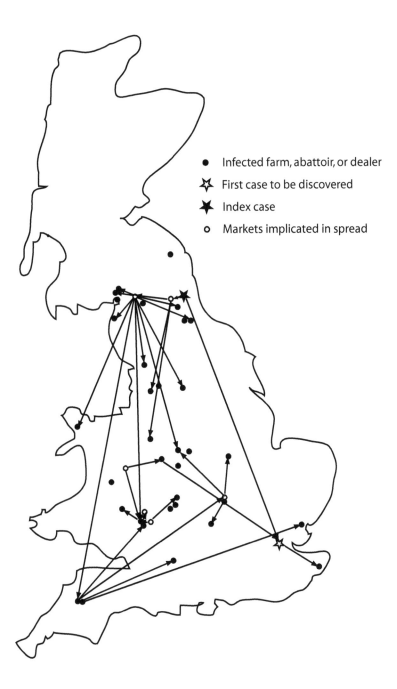

Figure 7.1 The early spread of the 2001 U.K. foot-and-mouth disease epidemic.
Adapted from Davies (2002), Figure 1.

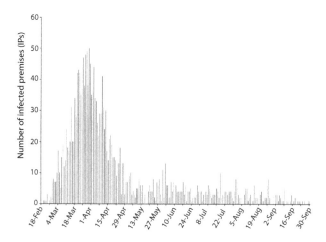

Figure 7.2 Epidemic curve showing daily cases of foot-and-mouth disease during the 2001 U.K. epidemic. Original source: Department of Environment, Food and Rural Affairs (DEFRA), U.K.

implications. One major difference between the two epidemics, however, was that in 2001, in addition to using traditional epidemiological methods to attempt to control the epidemic, authorities took the unusual step of inviting mathematical modelers to devise models to assess different control strategies at the time the epidemic was occurring. Results from these models were used to support controversial policies directed at control of the epidemic. The epidemic began to decline soon after the policies were implemented, but it is still not clear how strong a role the modeling activities actually played in this decline.

FMD only infects animals other than humans, but its impact on humans is significant, both in terms of economic costs and also in terms of its effects on social interactions, politics, and other spheres of human existence. For example, although the total costs of the 2001 U.K. epidemic are not completely known, estimates are that costs to the food and farming sectors of the country reached nearly $5 billion, the costs to the leisure and tourism industries were almost as high, and there were an additional $3 billion in other costs as well (Kitching et al., 2005; Thompson et al., 2002). Access was restricted to the public rights of way used extensively by recreational walkers and for the next year people were advised to stay away from infected areas (which included one of the most heavily used hiking areas in the U.K.). These policies caused serious problems in the many affected regions where tourism and recreation were nearly as important as farming to the economy (Mort et al., 2005). Studies focusing on the health effects of the U.K. epidemic and a concurrent epidemic in the Netherlands indicated that a large proportion of farmers and workers in the tourism industry experienced severe enough post-traumatic stress syndrome to require medical treatment, and the extent of these problems was clearly correlated to the severity of the epidemic within a region (Hannay and Jones, 2002; Olff et al., 2005).

The 2001 U.K. FMD epidemic was also clearly tied to the geographic structure of farms within the U.K. as well as factors structuring the social interactions of different animals within and among farms. These factors are also critical in understanding the geographic spread of diseases specific to human populations, and the kinds of approaches used to study the FMD epidemic are analogous to those used for many human diseases. In addition, because of the economic importance of domesticated animals, detailed records were (and still are) kept of where and when livestock were transported from one location to another, thereby providing essential data needed for effective geographic modeling. As discussed in the chapter on influenza models, such data are rarely available for human populations. Diseases such as FMD thus provide exceptional opportunities for exploring how well geographic models capture the local and regional details of epidemic spread across space and how useful such models are in controlling that spread.

The 2001 U.K. FMD epidemic is one of the most interesting examples of how mathematical models can help to guide policy-making and epidemic control strategies in response to an emergency situation, but it also clearly illustrates some of the difficulties associated with bringing models into play in a policy-making role. The remainder of this chapter briefly describes the models that were used, the control strategies that were implemented as a consequence of model results, and the response to these policies, especially from the veterinary epidemiological community. We also discuss criticisms of those strategies in the immediate aftermath of the epidemic and additional modeling work that was stimulated by those criticisms and other analyses of the overall impact of the implemented strategies. We close with comments on the use of models during this epidemic and lessons to be learned from the experience.

7.1 MODELING THE GEOGRAPHIC SPREAD OF FMD

Foot-and-mouth disease is caused by multiple strains of a highly contagious virus, with different strains predominating in different regions
of the world. The virus can persist in the environment for a month
or more in damp soil, especially under cold conditions. Plumes of
virus can be ejected in droplets into the air from the coughs of infected animals and then dispersed by wind over long distances (Gloster
et al., 1981; Hugh-Jones and Wright, 1970). The virus infects cloven-
footed mammals, including cattle, sheep, goats, and pigs in Europe
and camel and buffalo in neighboring regions (Moutou and Durand,
1994). Figure 7.3 summarizes the disease progression and relevant
epidemiology of foot-and-mouth disease. The severity of the disease
and the duration of infection vary among the different host animals,
with sheep being less seriously affected than cattle or pigs. Most
animals recover, but they may show permanently reduced weight or
milk yield, and mortality in young animals can be very high (Ferguson et al., 2001a). A vaccine for the disease is available, but the
immunization takes several days to induce immunity and may only
last for a few months. Furthermore, vaccinated animals may still be
susceptible and may develop subclinical infection that can be passed
on to other animals (Cox et al., 1999; Doel et al., 1994; Salt et al.,
1998; Woolhouse and Donaldson, 2001), which can have a significant
influence on the relative effectiveness of different control strategies.

A number of models have been developed to describe the spread of
FMD, including most recently Bates et al. (2003a,c), Ferguson et al.
(2001a,b), Kao (2003), Keeling et al. (2001, 2003), Matthews et al.
(2003), Morris et al. (2001), Rivas et al. (2003), and Sorensen et al.
(2000). The discussion below centers on the models of Ferguson, Keeling, and Morris and their colleagues, since these were the models used
to guide official policy during the 2001 U.K. epidemic.

Many factors contribute to the spread of FMD across space, with
perhaps the most important of these the spatial distribution of farms,
the connections between different farms (especially through movement of animals, people, or vehicles), the geographic distance between
farms, and the number and types of animals at each farm. FMD is a
contagious disease and spreads directly from one animal to another,
but because the focus of modeling efforts during the 2001 epidemic
was on local and regional geographic spread and because data were
often collated at the farm or higher level, the three models developed
during the course of that epidemic used farms rather than individuals
as the unit of transmission. Whenever possible model parameters for

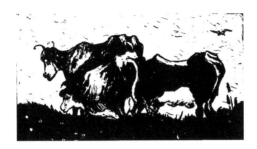

Infection occurs through contact with infected animals, foodstuffs, or other objects contaminated by infected animals, or by eating or coming into contact with infected carcasses; transmission between farms has been traced to movement of animals, persons, vehicles, and other objects; airborne transmission has also been observed

Incubation period of 2-14 days	Transmission can occur before symptoms are apparent

Development of fever, shivering, painful mouth, reduced milk yield with sores on teats of stock, lameness or tenderness of feet

Recovery occurs 8-15 days	after symptoms are apparent

Mortality is generally low, but disease can cause permanent reductions in milk yields, chronic lameness, sterility and higher rates of abortion, and other serious consequences; also, cattle may become carriers for 18-24 months following recovery

Figure 7.3 Essential elements of the disease progression and epidemiology of foot-and-mouth disease.

all three models were estimated using extensive data sets provided by British veterinary authorities.

Ferguson et al. (2001a,b) developed a deterministic compartmental model consisting of two components: 1) a traditional mass action transmission term to describe initial long-range contacts, and 2) a spatial correlation structure to allow the model to capture the structure of the contact network between neighboring farms and the more local transmission that dominated later transmission. The model was fitted to three sets of data on disease incidence — reports of cases, confirmation data, and notifications of slaughtering of animals. The initial model, which was described in Ferguson et al. (2001a), assumed that farms consisted of a single type of animal and that all farms had the same number of animals. This assumption was relaxed in Ferguson et al. (2001b) — the species mix, animal numbers, and number of distinct land parcels within farms were identified as important risk factors determining spatiotemporal patterns.

Keeling et al. (2001) developed an individual farm-based stochastic model of the epidemic. Individual farms were considered the epidemiological units and were classified as either susceptible, incubating, infectious, or slaughtered. Heterogeneity in farm size and species composition were incorporated by allowing susceptibility and infectiousness to vary with the number of animals present and the relative proportions of different livestock species. Local and regional spatial clustering of FMD cases were represented by a spatial infection kernel, which designated a high probability of local spread with a tail of less frequent long-range infections. Keeling et al. recognized two important features of the outbreak that needed to be captured by the model: 1) marked variability in daily case reports, and 2) an unusually long epidemic tail. They postulated that the first was likely to be due to stochastic effects, while the second was primarily related to the spatial nature of the infection. Because of the probable importance of stochastic and spatial effects, they chose to use a spatially structured stochastic model in their analysis of the epidemic and potential control methods.

The third model used to describe the 2001 U.K. epidemic was a spatial Monte Carlo simulation model of FMD called InterSpread that was developed in the early 1990s by Sanson and colleagues (1999). This model has been progressively refined and generalized since that time and was applied to the 2001 epidemic by Morris et al. (2001). It has also been adapted to model classical swine fever and other diseases of domesticated animals (Jalvingh et al., 1999; Nielen et al., 1999). The model set up a simulated group of farms that were popu-

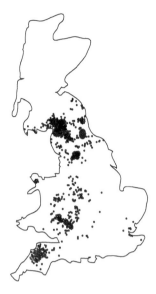

Figure 7.4 The spatial distribution of affected farms during the 2001 U.K. foot-and-mouth epidemic. Adapted from Gibbens et al. (2001), Figure 1.

lated with domesticated animals. Rather than using a distribution of spatial distances among farms to represent contact, the model explicitly incorporated the movement of animals, personnel, and vehicles, and also included wind-borne transmission. Infectivity was allowed to vary both according to the stage of the disease process on a farm and as a consequence of the implementation of control measures. In addition, a set of transmission parameters were used to govern how the disease spread among farms.

Local spatial structure was clearly an important feature of disease transmission during this epidemic. Infected farms were highly clustered in time and space (Figure 7.4) and in many cases transmission between farms could be linked directly to transport of infected animals, people, or vehicles (Gibbens et al., 2001). Both the Keeling model and the Morris model incorporated detailed structures based on knowledge about the known locations of the farms at risk. Such structures can result in time-consuming and costly simulations and, in addition, general mathematical descriptions are not possible. The Ferguson model, on the other hand, did not explicitly incorporate spatial structure; rather, it used a moment closure analytical technique that was conceptually more difficult, but perhaps simpler to implement (Kao, 2002).

The three models also differed in the way they handled heterogeneity in the composition of different farms. The deterministic structure of the Ferguson model necessitated significant simplifications in how the farms were conceived. The initial Ferguson model assumed that the distribution of animals did not vary among farms; their second model assumed the distribution varied, but did not explicitly model individual farm composition. Variation among farms was taken into account by separating the farms into four general classes (cattle, sheep, pig, and small farms under 100 animals), determining the class by most prevalent species, and allowing the transmission coefficient, the culling hazard, and the neighborhood size estimate to vary with the class of farm. Both the Keeling and Morris models identified and kept track of individual farms and were better able to handle interfarm heterogeneities. The Keeling model used only a few essential parameters to characterize farms, including the number and species of individual animals and species-specific transmission rates and susceptibilities. The Morris model was much more detailed, and incorporated 54 different parameters, including, for example, number of different low-, medium-, and high-risk movements of animals to different locations, parameters for airborne spread, proportions of lactating cattle at dairy farms, and number of dairy tanker pickups per week.

The focus of all three models was on evaluating the effectiveness of different potential control policies to help curb the epidemic. Policies curtailing the movement of animals were an immediate and standard response to reports of the disease; hence, all models incorporated this response as a basic structure (in other words, all variations in control strategies included movement control plus some other strategy). Traditional control strategies also involve disinfection of infected properties and rapid slaughter of animals not only at premises with an infected animal (IPs), but also at premises with documented contacts with an IP (these contacts are referred to as "dangerous contacts" and so such premises are called DCs) (Haydon et al., 2004). Additional strategies addressed by the models included both these traditional approaches and other options proposed by government advisory groups, the most controversial of which involved slaughter of animals at farms adjacent to infected farms (contiguous premises or CPs) regardless of whether infection had been detected at such farms. In particular, the strategies evaluated by the modelers included slaughter of all animals at infected premises, usually within 24 hours (IP culling), IP culling plus slaughter at contiguous premises within 48 or 72 hours (CP culling), IP culling plus slaughter targeted at premises with known (dangerous) contacts with infected premises (DC culling), ring vaccination (vaccination of all animals within a certain distance from an IP), targeted vaccination (vaccination of animals at high-risk premises), and a variety of combined approaches. Modeling was used to explore the impacts of qualitatively different approaches (e.g., DC culling vs. CP culling), the effects of various delays in implementing control strategies, and the value of multiple vs. single control strategies.

Despite their different structures and modeling approaches, these models all came to the same general conclusions, although the deterministic model was unable to capture the irregular behavior in the epidemic tail, and therefore did not provide good predictions of the final outcome of the epidemic. All models pointed out that control of the disease required effective movement restrictions and culling of animals not only on affected, but also on neighboring farms. They suggested that the most effective use of resources would be to speed up the time between diagnosis and culling and to focus on neighborhood culling. Model results generated during the epidemic also suggested that vaccination alone would not be of much use in disease control, and, furthermore, the effects of vaccination in combination with neighborhood culling were nearly indistinguishable from those of neighborhood culling alone.

7.2   THE OFFICIAL RESPONSE TO THE EPIDEMIC AND ITS AFTERMATH

As a consequence of the epidemiological modeling results, in late March 2001 the U.K. government formally confirmed a controversial policy involving IP culling within 24 hours and CP culling within 48 hours, without waiting for verification of high-risk status on the CPs. Additional culling of animals on farms within 3 km of an infected premise was recommended for heavily infected areas, but this latter policy was only implemented in Scotland (Bickerstaff and Simmons, 2004; Davies, 2002). Vaccination was also discussed as an option, but a decision was made not to incorporate this strategy, primarily because of the already widespread nature of the epidemic. The world then watched as an estimated 6 million animals were slaughtered (Bickerstaff and Simmons, 2004), destroying the livelihoods of numerous farmers as well as strongly affecting the tourism industry in one of the most heavily visited regions of the country.

One major reason mathematical modelers were called in to assess the value of different control measures is that predictions of the potential spread of the epidemic were dire. Early estimates predicted the epidemic would last many months, might result in more than 4000 outbreaks a day by June 2001, and might double in size every 8 days (Davies, 2002). The ultimate costs of such a devastating epidemic would have been enormous and had such an epidemic occurred, those costs would likely have been more than even the massive costs that actually came to pass.

In reality, the 2001 FMD epidemic began to wane shortly after the model-informed culling policy was implemented, and, in fact, aggregated national level data appeared to indicate that the decline of the epidemic coincided with the onset of high levels of CP culling (Honhold et al., 2004). This led to claims that the strategy resulting from the modeling efforts played a major role in controlling an epidemic that was threatening to rapidly spiral out of control (see, for example, Ferguson et al., 2001a; Woolhouse, 2003). Data analyzed at a finer geographic scale suggest, however, that the onset of high levels of CP culling was not necessarily closely linked to the timing of the epidemic (Honhold et al., 2004). In addition, even at the time the CP culling policy was initiated, there were many disagreements about the actual value of the models and the policy based on them, and in the years since the epidemic several substantive critiques of the official responses to the epidemic have been published (e.g., Bates et al., 2003b; Green and Medley, 2002; Haydon et al., 2004; Honhold et al., 2004; Kao, 2002; Keeling, 2005; Kitching et al., 2005, 2006; Moutou, 2002; Thrusfield et al., 2005; Woolhouse, 2003). Criticisms center primarily around three issues: 1) whether the models were adequate representations of reality, 2) whether the contiguous cull policy was truly beneficial, and 3) whether traditional epidemiological approaches would have been adequate in the absence of the additional contiguous culling.

The question of whether models are adequate representations of reality comes up with nearly every modeling attempt and is inherent in the modeling process. Models always involve simplifying assumptions, and, as such, arguments can always be made about their applicability to the real world. Development of the three major FMD models proceeded with full knowledge of these limitations, however, and in order to minimize potential problems from necessary simplifications, the models were validated using data of the highest quality possible. This process indicated that the models were robust and convinced authorities that results of model simulations were adequate to inform official policy at the time of the epidemic given the perceived urgency of the situation.

Nonetheless, analyses after the epidemic died out have pointed out several issues that should be taken into account in the future. The most serious of these issues relate to adequacy of the data used to estimate model parameters and/or support model assumptions. Although the models were based on the best data available, they were inadequate in a number of dimensions that could have had a strong impact on the policies recommended to the authorities. For example, there was significant uncertainty in the estimates of infectiousness available to the modelers (Haydon et al., 2004). In particular, there was inadequate information on the relative proportion of subclinical (and hence unrecognized) cases. It has been proposed that estimates used during the epidemic severely underestimated the number of subclinical cases, which resulted in overestimates of the transmission probability and led to predictions of more rapid epidemic spread than were perhaps realistic (Kitching et al., 2005). The models also assumed that the distance between farms was the main determinant of risk, but the state of scientific knowledge of the disease was not adequate to determine if this was the case. Although such an assumption was a logical one to make, it would bias results in favor of the contiguous culling policy that was implemented because that policy was directly based on the distance between farms. Some analyses of the sensitivity of model results to these assumptions was performed, but uncertainty remains about whether these sensitivity analyses were adequate at the time policies were implemented (Haydon et al., 2004). It must be kept in mind, however, that authorities were dealing with what was perceived to be an emergency situation. In emergencies decisions are sometimes made that, in hindsight, may not have been the absolute best, but humans are not omniscient, so one must be cautious about placing undue blame after the fact.

The latter two issues, about whether the contiguous cull policy was truly beneficial and whether traditional epidemiological approaches would have been adequate, are fundamentally linked to one another, and the answers to those questions are still a matter of much controversy. Thrusfield et al. (2005) proposed that, at least in some areas, culls of healthy animals that were designed to limit spread (pre-emptive culls) may have actually begun after the epidemic had already peaked. This assessment depends on the date used for the epidemic peak, however, and there is some disagreement about this date. Kitching et al. (2005) assert that the peak occurred on March 27, Gibbens et al. (2001) state that the peak was reached on March 26, but stayed at that level for the next week, while others claim an early

April peak (e.g., Davies, 2002). A further issue is that the connection between the epidemic peak and the implementation of contiguous culling is apparent when looking at data aggregated at the national level, but as mentioned above, this may not have been the case at finer geographic scales. As Honhold et al. (2004) point out, differences in the relative numbers of different animal species as well as differences in the application of control measures in different regions indicate substantial geographic heterogeneity. Thus, separate analyses in different regions are probably necessary to assess how effective the contiguous cull policy was in actually controlling the epidemic, especially in consideration of the fact that traditional techniques worked reasonably well in earlier epidemics of the disease (Haydon et al., 2004).

The disastrous consequences of the 2001 FMD epidemic have caused the European and U.K. veterinary public health communities to devote substantial energy towards developing better policies and strategies to use when faced with the next major epidemic. In particular, the 2003 European Union Directive and the U.K.'s 2004 FMD contingency plans have recommended that reactive vaccination be used as a preferred means of intervention during future outbreaks, although the plans did not specify particular designs for the programs (Tildesley et al., 2006). Because of this, new modeling studies have been conducted to help assess the relative value of different proposed designs.

The first of these studies was that of Keeling et al. (2003), who used their individual-based model developed during the epidemic itself (Keeling et al., 2001) to further explore the potential effectiveness of different control strategies. Analysis of a number of different vaccination scenarios led them to modify the conclusions of their earlier work. Their new work indicated that, particularly if the vaccination strategies were to take advantage of the spatial structure of at-risk farms, both prophylactic and reactive vaccination strategies could prove effective in controlling epidemics. They noted a number of uncertainties that could be important for any particular epidemic, however, including economic issues, farming practices, the lag between uptake of the vaccination and generation of immunity, the need to have full cooperation from farmers, and logistic and practical difficulties. Nonetheless, their work showed how attention to detailed spatial information can dramatically affect conclusions about the potential for different control strategies to affect the patterns of spread of infectious diseases across heterogeneous landscapes.

In an elaboration of this work, Tildesley et al. (2006) used the same model of FMD spread, but focused on the strategy of ring vaccination and the logistical constraints that might be present during an epidemic and that might cause real strategies to vary from an ideal policy. Ring vaccination involves determination of minimum and maximum distances that define a ring surrounding a particular IP. All farms that occur within that ring are then targeted for the vaccination campaign. Tildesley et al. assumed that priority for vaccination would be based on the order in which affected IPs were reported, and if two or more farms were identified on the same day, then the farm furthest from the IP would take precedence, leading to a strategy whereby vaccination would move from the outside of the ring to the inside. They also assumed that only cattle were vaccinated, that the vaccine was 90% effective, and that it would take about 4 days for vaccine-induced immunity to take effect. Results of this model indicated that CP culling would be successful in the absence of vaccination, but would not be advantageous if combined with vaccination. Tildesley et al. (2006) also found that using proximity to a previously infected premise as the basis for determining vaccination priority was a simple and successful strategy that did not require additional knowledge about the optimal size of the ring used to identify at-risk farms.

As was the case with the initial FMD models during the 2001 outbreak, the results of these models addressing vaccination strategies have been called into question by members of the veterinary public health community. These critiques have resulted in a lively discussion in the literature (see, for example, Wingfield et al. (2006) and Kitching et al. (2007) and the corresponding responses by Keeling et al. (2006) and Tildesley et al. (2007)), which promises to continue for some time and clearly indicates the difficulties inherent in attempts to combine mathematical modeling insights with real-world situations.

In general, mathematical models have also ignored a very important issue that clearly impacted the entire 2001 FMD experience. In particular, the modeling efforts ignored the economic and social impacts of the different control policies. The official decision to adopt a contiguous cull policy led to the slaughter of a huge number of healthy animals who may have been at fairly low risk for the disease and resulted in large-scale economic and social disruption that extended long after the epidemic was over. This lack of attention to the relative costs and benefits of the proposed policies is unfortunate, but again, it is important to recognize that this does not justify exclusion of mathematical approaches when faced with large-scale epidemics.

The questions of whether the contiguous cull policy adopted during the 2001 epidemic was truly beneficial and what might be the best control strategies to pursue in the future have still not been answered definitively and will probably continue to be discussed for decades to come. Although it is possible that the 2001 epidemic would have subsided using traditional epidemiological strategies without the CP culling policy, there is no way to know for sure whether that would have been the case. Rather, the controversy points to the crucial need for regular communication between 1) traditional epidemiologists, who have first-hand and direct experience with the individuals most affected by a disease, 2) mathematical modelers, who have new and valuable technological methods to bring into play, and 3) policy makers, who have the resources and authority to make things happen. The most important lesson to be learned from the experience with the 2001 U.K. FMD epidemic is that major epidemics impact society in a multitude of ways, and so this kind of communication will help to guarantee that the strategy chosen for the next major epidemic is epidemiologically sound, cost-effective, and sensitive to the social and economic needs of the people most affected by the epidemic. Mathematical models are a new tool to use to help in making control decisions, but they must be used in conjunction with the input of a variety of other disciplines in order to maximize their advantages and minimize their limitations.

Chapter Eight

Maps, Projections, and GIS:

Geographers' Approaches

When most people think of how objects, entities, or characteristics are distributed in and spread across space, they think of geography and maps. Yet much of the work of geographers on the spatial spread of infectious diseases is relatively unknown within the epidemic modeling community. Geographers have been studying the spread of infectious diseases across space for some time, however, and they have developed a number of methods for attacking this question. Many of their approaches draw primarily upon statistical analyses of spatial data rather than the development of mechanistic mathematical models, but a few investigators have used mathematical models in conjunction with other types of geographical analyses. In this chapter we introduce many of the most common techniques geographers have used, with special emphasis on the kinds of questions addressed and the value of geographic approaches in answering those questions. Readers interested in learning the details of how to implement specific techniques are encouraged to consult textbooks on spatial analysis, such as Cliff and Haggett (1988) or Haining (2003).

8.1 MAPPING METHODS

One of the essential components in a geographer's study of disease spread is a map. Maps have been around since the beginning of recorded history (and probably were present much earlier), but cartographic methods focused on answering particular scientific questions did not get their start until around 1800 (Walter, 2000). Maps to describe the geographic spread of infectious diseases have been a valuable aid to visualizing patterns across time and space. Figure 8.1 gives several examples of simple kinds of maps used to study the geographic spread of infectious diseases.

Most mapping techniques are focused on smoothing data to simplify the picture and bring important features to the forefront. The goal is to separate the broad trends that form a signal in the data from the noise or local variability surrounding those trends, much as a radio tuner isolates the emitted signal from a particular station (Cliff and Haggett, 1988). Major approaches used for this purpose include spatial filtering or averaging, trend surface analysis, kriging, and Bayesian approaches.

In spatial filtering the points to be used in deriving the map are based on a simple or weighted average of points in the region being considered plus surrounding regions. Weighting functions can take a variety of forms and are chosen so that they smooth out fluctuations between regions and minimize the effects of random variability. This strategy was used by Gould et al. (1991) to study the spatial spread of HIV in Pennsylvania and by Gardner et al. (1989) to study the spread of HIV among military recruits in four urban areas of the United States. Maps resulting from this method often use shading to represent the hills and valleys in the levels of disease across a landscape (see Figure 8.4).

Trend surface analysis is probably the most commonly used mapping technique within geography and consists of finding a polynomial surface that best fits a set of points to be mapped. The resulting map looks something like a topographic map that might be used by hikers to help plan their route. Angulo et al. (1977) used this technique to map the spread of a variola minor epidemic in Brazil. The dates of introduction of the disease into households formed the primary data set used in generating these maps, and the resulting contours represented when, on average, the epidemic reached particular areas (Figure 8.2). Trend surface analysis was also essentially the basis for maps produced by Löytönen and colleagues in their studies of the spread of HIV in Finland and Puerto Rico (Löytönen, 1991, 1994; Löytönen and Arbona, 1996; Löytönen and Maasilta, 1997), although they were usually represented as 3-dimensional surfaces or as vertical bars extending up from a 2-dimensional base map of the country involved rather than as 2-dimensional contour maps.

Spatial filtering and trend surface analysis have two major limitations (Carrat and Valleron, 1992). First, these techniques usually do not take full advantage of the spatial structure of a variable. Second, the methods do not allow one to estimate the degree of error of the interpolations. To deal with these limitations, Carrat and Valleron proposed that geographers use kriging, a technique first developed in the earth sciences. Kriging produces a model that describes the spatial dependence between samples and is not constrained by the borders of the geographic units of analysis. It results in a continu-

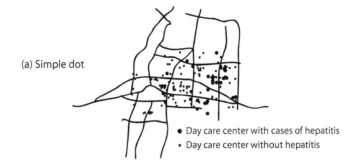

(a) Simple dot

● Day care center with cases of hepatitis
· Day care center without hepatitis

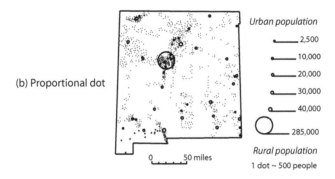

(b) Proportional dot

Urban population

2,500
10,000
20,000
30,000
40,000
285,000

0   50 miles

Rural population
1 dot ~ 500 people

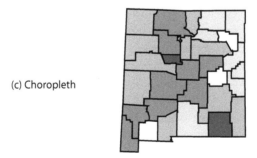

(c) Choropleth

Figure 8.1 Examples of mapping techniques used to visualize disease patterns across time and space. a) Simple dot map showing presence or absence of hepatitis A in Albuquerque, New Mexico day care centers during a 1984 epidemic. b) Proportional dot map indicating relative population sizes of New Mexico towns and cities, 1978. Data from the U.S. Bureau of the Census, 1978. c) Choropleth map, which uses different shades to represent the relative frequency of hepatitis A cases in New Mexico counties, 1979. Each county is filled with a uniform color that indicates its hepatitis frequency. White areas reported no cases; darker shades indicate higher frequency. Data from the New Mexico Communicable Disease Survey, 1979. Directed graphs are also a type of map; see Figure 2.5.

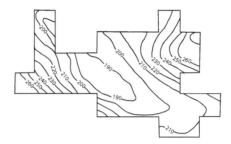

Figure 8.2 Cubic trend surface analysis map of the spread of variola minor among
            households in a Brazilian community. Redrawn from Angulo et al.
            (1977).

ous map that avoids sudden transitions between regions. Because it
is continuous, missing data can be filled in using existing data from
neighboring sampled points. Carrat and Valleron illustrated the technique with data on the geographic distribution of an influenza-like
illness in France. The resulting maps look very much like contour
maps produced using trend surface analysis and show the epidemic's
temporal spread across the country.

Assunção et al. (2001) advocated the use of Bayesian approaches
to smooth maps of disease distributions. Their approach imposed a
plausible spatial structure on the region and used that structure in
modeling the relative risks for disease across a region. Thus, like the
kriging method, information on areas surrounding a region of interest
was used to improve the estimation of the region being considered.
Assunção et al. (2001) stated that Bayesian maps are smoother than
crude rate maps that have been based on maximum likelihood estimates, and they give rise to maps that are more informative visually
and easier to interpret. They also used Bayesian approaches to predict the space-time spread of human visceral leishmaniasis in Brazil.
Their statistical approach was used to generate predicted values for
disease rates in the different zones of a Brazilian city. They then designed a shading scheme for the range of variation in these values and
shaded each zone according to its projected rate of disease (a similar
technique was also used for the observed data). This generated a map
that was visually similar to the choropleth map shown in Figure 8.1c.

The majority of mapping studies are primarily descriptive and retrospective and do not go beyond that level, although Assunção et al.

(2001) is a notable exception. New statistical techniques have been developed to adjust and smooth data to make better maps, but they are still generally descriptive and retrospective and have limited predictive capabilities. The bulk of modeling work in medical geography, on the other hand, has used maps as a tool to help understand how and why geographic patterns have come about. A substantial percentage of this work has concentrated on the analysis of spatial heterogeneity at a particular time, with little attention paid to changes in the spatial distribution over time. Or, when the time dimension is explicitly considered, analysis of the spatial pattern itself is often limited to an informal discussion of observed patterns (Walter, 2000). Analysis of the space-time distribution of infectious diseases is a growing area within medical geography, however, and is the focus of the rest of this chapter.

Most of the statistical techniques that have been used in a space-time context (as opposed to a purely spatial or purely temporal context) center on three types of questions: identifying broad patterns of disease diffusion, projecting the future spread of epidemics, and detecting spatio-temporal disease clusters and spatial heterogeneity. These are all important questions to address in studies of the geographic spread of infectious diseases, but they have received varying degrees of attention by geographers. The majority of work focuses on identifying broad patterns of disease spread across space, both in modern populations and in historical populations. Detecting disease clusters and spatial heterogeneity is a rapidly growing area of interest, especially with the advent of geographic information systems (GIS) technology.[1] Projecting the future spatial spread of epidemics, although perhaps of greatest importance from a practical point of view, has received less attention within geography than the other two areas.

8.2 IDENTIFYING PATTERNS OF DISEASE DIFFUSION

Geographers commonly consider three broad categories of diffusion: spatially contagious diffusion, hierarchical diffusion, and transfer or relocation diffusion. Spatially contagious diffusion (also referred to as contact diffusion) is diffusion that occurs as a result of direct contact between neighboring regions (Cliff et al., 1981; Meade and Earickson,

---

[1]GIS systems are a sophisticated way to capture, store, retrieve, and display spatial data. They include both data of interest (e.g., disease prevalences, environmental features, or density of mosquitoes or humans) and spatial information, as well as a means to link such data together.

2000). This type of diffusion appears to spread out from its point of introduction in a wave-like pattern and shows a strong distance effect, with the probability of transmission between regions declining with increasing distance (Figure 8.3a). Hierarchical diffusion is characterized by transmission among urban, suburban, and rural areas according to their relative size. Typically, the point of introduction of a disease characterized by such spread is a large urban center, from which it spreads to secondary centers of population, and then to still smaller communities, and into the hinterland. The diffusion process appears to follow a branching type structure (Figure 8.3b). Spatially contagious diffusion and hierarchical diffusion are subcategories of a more general pattern called expansion diffusion, which is characterized by expansion of a phenomenon (e.g., a disease, idea, or technological advance) out from a central place (or places) in a relatively smooth fashion. The third major diffusion pattern, called transfer diffusion by Smallman-Raynor and Cliff (2001a) or relocation diffusion by Cliff et al. (1981) and Meade and Earickson (2000), results when the phenomenon that is spreading jumps over some distance from the area of origin to a new location (Figure 8.3c). This can occur because of the nature of modern global transportation patterns, or because of large-scale population relocations associated with troop movements during wars, refugees fleeing oppressive or dangerous conditions, or similar events.

Determination of the relative importance of each of these patterns within a region can aid in developing strategies for the control of infectious disease spread that take advantage of natural patterns of interaction. For example, ring vaccination strategies are likely to be more effective when the predominant diffusion pattern is spatially contagious, since the vaccination barrier can completely surround the area of active disease transmission. On the other hand, if relocation diffusion is prominent, ring vaccination will be less effective since there is a significant probability of jumps to regions outside the vaccination area.

Both cartographic and statistical methods are used to analyze patterns of disease spread across a landscape. One of the simplest cartographic methods is the construction of a set of maps that represent the relative disease risks across the landscape at a series of times (Figure 8.4). (This method is broadly similar to the technique used in magnetic resonance imaging to produce a three-dimensional view of the inside of the body.) Successive maps can then be compared to identify the location of new or persistent outbreaks and determine the pattern of spread of the epidemic through a community or region.

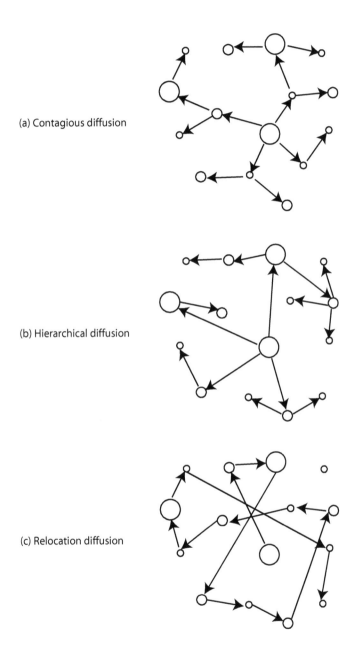

(a) Contagious diffusion

(b) Hierarchical diffusion

(c) Relocation diffusion

Figure 8.3 Types of diffusion patterns. See text for a description of the major characteristics of each.

A second method is to use qualitative accounts to draw vector maps of the spread of an epidemic, with arrows showing the direction and often the magnitude of spread throughout a region. See Cliff and Haggett (1988) for a more complete description of these and other cartographic methods for analyzing the space-time distribution of a disease.

No matter how a sequence of maps is derived, if the time dimension is measured explicitly, then it may be possible to calculate lag times between when a disease enters different communities and determine important characteristics of epidemic spread. For example, Cliff et al. (1981) analyzed data on the spread of measles in Iceland and determined that the average lag time was a function of population size and distance from the capital, Reykjavik, with the time increasing as population size decreased and distance increased. They also determined that population size was a more important determinant of the speed of disease diffusion than was distance.

To rigorously test the importance of spatially contagious, hierarchical, and relocation diffusion in explaining observed disease patterns, geographers use a variety of statistical and mathematical modeling approaches. These are probably easier to explain in the context of examples of studies that have been performed. Andrew Cliff and his colleagues, Peter Haggett, Keith Ord, Matthew Smallman-Raynor, and others, have been the most influential geographers in this area and have produced numerous books and papers analyzing epidemics for variety of diseases in several locations and different times. Smallman-Raynor and Cliff's analyses of an historical cholera epidemic on the Philippine Islands following the Philippine-American War (Smallman-Raynor and Cliff, 1998b,c, 2001b) will be used to illustrate many of the available methods. Although this work is centered on an historical epidemic, the methods used are appropriate for modern epidemics and the results serve to illustrate the kinds of insights that can be derived from such studies.

The cholera epidemic analyzed by Smallman-Raynor and Cliff began just as the Philippine war ended. It comprised two waves, one occurring from 22 March 1902 to 28 February 1903 and the other occurring from 16 May 1903 to 6 February 1904. Detailed data on the epidemic were gleaned from sanitary dispatches prepared by the Chief Quarantine Officer for the Philippine Islands and reprinted in the United States Public Health Service publication, *Public Health Reports*. Smallman-Raynor and Cliff (1998b) is an analysis of wave I data; Smallman-Raynor and Cliff (1998c) is an analysis of wave II data.

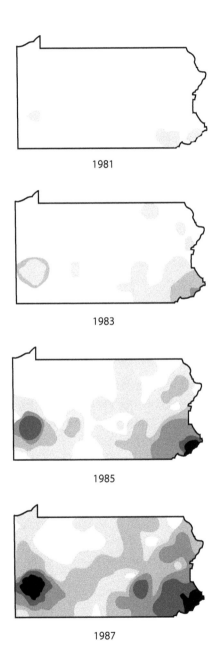

1981

1983

1985

1987

Figure 8.4 The spread of HIV across Pennsylvania between 1981 and 1987. Adapted from Gould et al. (1991), Figure 1.

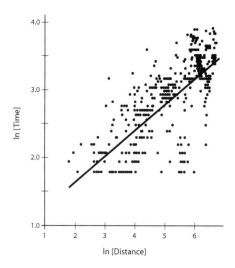

Figure 8.5 Relationship between the time of first appearance of cholera during a
1902-04 epidemic in the Philippines and distance from the epidemic
origin. The number and position of the dots are approximations of
data given in Smallman-Raynor and Cliff (1998b), Figure 4.

The wave I data, which were more detailed than the data from wave
II, were initially analyzed using stepwise multiple regression. In this
technique, independent variables are successively added to a model
(or one can start with all possible independent variables and remove
selected ones successively) until most of the variation in the dependent
variables is explained by the independent variables chosen or retained.
Results from this analysis showed a marked positive association between the distance from Manila and the time the disease reached an
area, which was an indication of spatially contagious spread (Figure
8.5). There was only weak evidence for hierarchical spread, however,
and this was true at all spatial scales, from country-wide to island and
province levels.

The multiple regression analysis was only able to suggest the relative importance of different patterns as a whole, but because disease
diffusion is a contagion process, the timing of cases is highly influenced
by the spatial relationships between locations. In real epidemics different types of diffusion may be important at different stages of an
epidemic process, but multiple regression analysis is unable to capture that temporal variation. For that reason, Smallman-Raynor and
Cliff (1998b) also used spatial autocorrelation analysis on their data,

a technique that assesses the correlation between variables in relation to their spatial location. This technique is able to determine the changing roles of different diffusion processes as an epidemic progresses. Their results suggested that at the national level the transmission process started through localized (spatially contagious) spread from Manila to nearest-neighbor settlements, but as the epidemic approached its peak, hierarchical spread became more important, and then the pattern reverted to purely contagious spread as the epidemic faded out. Island and province findings were broadly similar to national level findings, although there was no evidence that fadeout of the epidemic at those levels was associated with purely contagious spread; rather, hierarchical spread continued to play a small but measurable role, especially at the island level.

Analysis of wave II data indicated significant differences in how the epidemic spread at the later time compared to wave I. The results identified three regionally discrete cells, all of which were characterized by tight linkages between neighboring units within the region. This is in sharp contrast to the identification of one central region that initiated spread throughout the islands observed during wave I.

Autocorrelation on graphs was used to determine whether the differences in waves I and II over time were a result of differences in the underlying diffusion process. This technique allows statistical analysis of time series data while still retaining information about the spatial characteristics of the disease patterns (see Cliff and Haggett (1988) for details on this method). Results showed that contagious spread was statistically significant during all stages of both waves; however, its significance waned as the peak of wave I was reached and then it built up again towards the end of that wave, while it was important throughout most of wave II (Figure 8.6a). Results also suggested that the contagious process for wave I was more strongly structured than for wave II. Furthermore, the mechanisms that underpinned the spatial development of wave I began well before peak morbidity, while the mechanisms that underpinned wave II were synchronized with morbidity patterns. Smallman-Raynor and Cliff (1998c) suggest that these results may be due to the fact that large-scale population movements were a major outcome of the war and its immediate aftermath, while at the time of wave II, mobility patterns had settled back to the more normal peacetime situation. Results also suggest that hierarchical diffusion did not play much of a role during most of the epidemic (Figure 8.6b).

To examine further the validity of these conclusions, Smallman-Raynor and Cliff (2001a) used multidimensional scaling to visualize

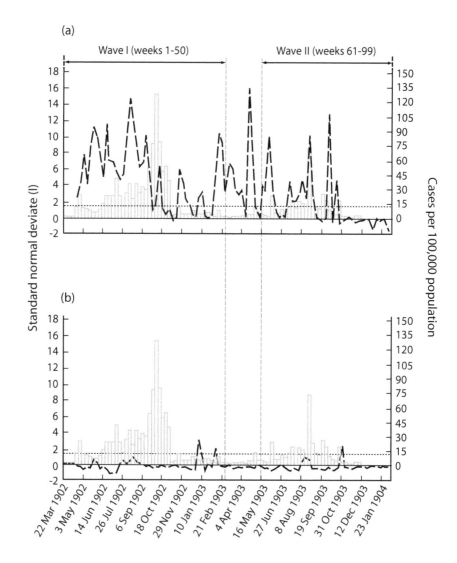

Figure 8.6 Autocorrelation graphs for the diffusion of cholera at the national level during the 1902-04 Philippines cholera epidemic. Gray bars plot the weekly cholera case rates, line graphs plot the weekly values of Moran's spatial autocorrelation coefficient, I, using a technique indicative of contagious spread (top graph) and one indicating hierarchical spread (bottom graph). Values of I above 1.65 (the dashed horizontal lines) indicate significant ($p < 0.05$) positive spatial autocorrelations and represent times when the actual diffusion process corresponded to the proposed pattern (contagious or hierarchical). Adapted from Smallman-Raynor and Cliff (1998c), Figure 4.

the epidemic and attempt to track the pathways by which it spread. This technique analyzes a data set to determine how close individual data points or groups within the data are to each other based on similarities among a number of variables in addition to or instead of geography. Essentially the goal is to arrange the data in a space of a dimension determined by the investigator. The "distances" between individuals or groups can then be explained in light of the variables that determined the chosen dimensions (e.g., on a road map the dimensions would be latitude vs. longitude; on a map of psychological space the dimensions might be extroversion/introversion on one axis and individualism/group behavior on the other). The analysis of Smallman-Raynor and Cliff (2001a) also indicated that the space (broadly defined) through which cholera diffused was fundamentally reorganized between the two cholera waves. As in the initial multiple regression, results of the multidimensional scaling indicated that the first wave emanated from a single location, Manila, while the second wave was associated with three distinct regional centers. Other results about the relative importance of different types of diffusion were also confirmed by multidimensional scaling.

Other examples of work of this type by Cliff, Smallman-Raynor, and colleagues include, for example, Cliff et al. (1981, 1983a, 1993), Cliff and Haggett (1985), and Smallman-Raynor and Cliff (1991, 1998a). In addition, a few other studies have focused on identifying the type of diffusion operating during an epidemic. Adesina (1984) looked at patterns of diffusion of a 1971 cholera epidemic in Ibadan City, Nigeria to determine which spatial processes were responsible for generating the observed data. Analyses indicated that the disease spread in an apparent wave-like fashion within a roughly circular area corresponding to the center of the old city. Lam et al. (1996) used spatial correlograms, which are diagrams showing changes in the spatial autocorrelations as a function of distance and time, to explore changes in yearly AIDS incidence rates by county for four regions in the United States between 1982 and 1990. They found that there was substantial regional heterogeneity and that most regions did not show patterns of diffusion that were readily explainable with standard models (i.e., contagious, hierarchical, or relocation diffusion). Golub et al. (1993) extended a compartmental epidemiological model for HIV transmission to include hierarchical and spatially contagious diffusion. They considered three spatial compartments in their model: the urban areas of their study region (Ohio), the rural areas of their study region, and the rest of the world. The model essentially assumed random mixing between compartments, did not divide the population into risk groups for the disease, and included several other simplifying assumptions. Diffusion was assumed to occur among the three compartments in a hierarchical fashion. Golub et al. (1993) found that the "spatial compartmental model fits observed AIDS incidence spatial diffusion patterns in Ohio reasonably well" (p. 85). This result is not surprising given the geographic scale they were considering and the lack of overall structure in the model — it is likely the model could fit many state-level sets of data reasonably well.

The results of all of these studies point out the primary uses of geographers' spatial analytic techniques and their value for understanding patterns of epidemic spread across space. They provide insights into how social events, settlement patterns, and contact among communities can influence broad disease diffusion patterns. These insights can be used to help design strategies for preparing for and controlling disease outbreaks, provided the setting upon which the analysis is based is not too different from the present situation. That leads, however, to the major question remaining in these kinds of studies — how generalizable are they? Unfortunately, there is no answer to this question yet, since the studies that have been done consider populations widely separated in time and space and a variety of diseases. What is ideally needed is a series of studies within at least two or three individual populations covering multiple epidemics of more than one disease over a time period of at least 25-50 years. Cliff and colleagues have addressed the spread of multiple diseases on the island of Iceland in a large number of studies, many of which have been described in this book. Additional similar studies in other locations would provide enough information on the potential variability in patterns of epidemic diffusion to be able to make reasonable generalizations that could be used in studies focused on predicting the characteristics of epidemics that are yet to occur.

8.3   EPIDEMIC PROJECTIONS

Projecting the future spatial spread of infectious diseases is clearly an important concern in determining adequate control strategies, but in this arena geographic approaches to the study of infectious diseases have probably experienced the least success. Primary reasons for this include an emphasis on either spatial diffusion or temporal change but not both, the relative lack of effective statistical and mathematical modeling methods available for space-time analyses and the complexity of those that are available, and a lack of adequate data with which to assess both spatial and temporal trends.

One of the additional problems associated with forecasting epidemics, both within and between populations, is that the size of the susceptible population changes over time, which may not be a problem in the early stages of a forecast, but which definitely becomes a factor as an epidemic progresses. In order to deal with this problem, Cliff and Ord (1978) developed a forecasting model based on a chain binomial model of disease transmission, a mathematical approach described in Chapter 2. Their results showed that the chain binomial model did not provide a good fit to either the data used in calibrating the model or the epidemic that was forecast by the model (Figure 8.7). They concluded that the chain binomial model was probably too simple to be of much use, so they abandoned it in much of their later work in favor of more statistically based nonmechanistic approaches. The work on predicting influenza epidemics of Baroyan and colleagues (e.g., Baroyan and Rvachev, 1978) and many other researchers could also be considered epidemic forecasting using a mathematical model as the basis, as could some of the uses of models during the 2001 U.K. foot-and-mouth disease epidemic. This work is discussed in more detail in the chapters on those diseases.

Most forecasting methods are based on statistical techniques that use a recent data set to project disease rates and patterns into the immediate future. For example, Cliff et al. (1983b) used logistic regression techniques to produce models of the way in which measles epidemics spread geographically on the island of Iceland. They then used their models to forecast the likely pathways along which future measles epidemics would move. The standard regression approach was adjusted to take into account both the lag between cases because of geographic distance between districts and the fact that the serial interval between natural transmissions of measles may be shorter than the data reporting interval, resulting in multiple steps in the chain of transmission within one reporting interval.

Cliff and Ord (1985) recognized that, because of the speed of epidemic spread for a disease like measles, accurate forecasts of the onset of an epidemic are at least as important as forecasts of later stages of spread. They developed a model that took into account not only the number of new cases in a month, but also reintroduction of the disease from outside after fadeout, and the fact that the probability of an epidemic depends on the number of susceptibles, which cannot generally be measured directly. Reintroduction of the disease was dealt with by basing a region's forecast on the number of cases in neighboring areas as well as on the number of cases within the region. The effect of number of susceptibles was handled by assuming that recruitment of new susceptibles was a linear function of time with periodic depletions during epidemics. Data from epidemics between January 1946 and December 1956 were used to derive the forecasting model, which was then used to make one-month-ahead predictions between January 1957 and December 1968. Comparisons between the forecasted model and actual data from 1956-68 showed that the results of their forecasts were mixed — some aspects of real epidemics were captured well by the model, others were not detected.

In a series of papers, Löytönen developed a forecasting model to predict the geographic spread of HIV in Finland (Löytönen, 1991, 1994; Löytönen and Maasilta, 1997) and in Puerto Rico (Löytönen and Arbona, 1996). Because of inadequate data, the HIV positive population was estimated by fitting past incidence figures to a number of standard curves (e.g., the logistic and Gompertz functions) and this estimated population was distributed over defined districts within the country. Correlation analysis and multiple stepwise regression were performed on a number of sociological, demographic, and epidemiological variables to derive a probability surface governing the risk of transmission in different regions, and then a Monte Carlo simulation was used to model the spread of the epidemic across the country. Results of the forecasting indicated that spread of the disease within Finland would likely follow a hierarchical pattern from urban centers to small cities to rural areas. Löytönen (1994) suggested that this might be reasonably valid for other stable industrialized countries with developed communications systems, but that less developed countries or those suffering from low intensity political conflicts might follow a different path. To test this hypothesis, Löytönen and Arbona (1996) used the same procedure to forecast the spread of HIV in Puerto Rico. They concluded that their model provided reasonable predictions of short-term diffusion on the island, but expressed a number of caveats related to 1) the nature of the data (which consisted of case reports rather than HIV status), 2) the impact of the long incubation period of the disease, and 3) the presence of significant interactions between Puerto Rican residents and U.S. Puerto Rican communities, an activity that was not included in the model. The number of caveats suggests that the generalization about disease diffusion patterns in different countries is probably too broad to hold up in practice.

Three other forecasting models deserve brief mention. Williams and Rees (1994) used a multiregional demographic projection model to predict the spatial and temporal diffusion of HIV within the U.K. Their model included almost all types of risk structures and behav-

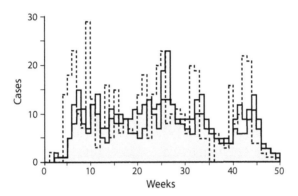

a) Calibration period

b) Forecast

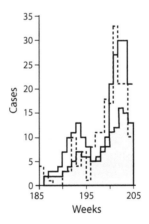

Figure 8.7 Calibration of a measles forecasting model and the resulting forecast. Top graph shows observed measles data (dashed line) and best-fit versions of a chain binomial model (solid line) and an exponential smoothing model (gray area). Bottom graph shows the observed data from a subsequent epidemic and the forecasts of that epidemic from the chain binomial and exponentially smoothed models. Adapted from Cliff and Ord (1978), Figure 12.2.

iors that had been determined to affect transmission of the disease, including three major transmission routes (sexual, needle-sharing, and perinatal), variable infectivity, behavior change, age-dependent patterns of sexual activity, and mobility at national and international levels. Results of their projections were pretty general and probably related to the incorporation of so many factors, many of which are not well understood. Gould et al. (1991) used spatial filtering (described briefly above) to predict a map of the future distribution of HIV in Pennsylvania, but their projections were at such a broad scale that they gave only a general picture of the course of the disease (see Figure 8.4). Finally, as also discussed briefly above, Assunção et al. (2001) used a space-time Bayesian estimation procedure in their study of visceral leishmaniasis in Brazil. Although their main focus was to analyze the degree of spatial heterogeneity, they went beyond simple description of the heterogeneity and developed projections of the future course of the disease based on Bayesian estimation procedures. They suggested that the information their models contributed about the relative risks for visceral leishmaniasis expected in different parts of the city would help to better direct control strategies to where they would be most effective.

8.4   DETECTION OF DISEASE CLUSTERING

A growing body of research centers on detecting clusters of disease in time and space or on determining how levels of heterogeneity in prevalence, incidence, or risk vary across the landscape. Determining the presence of unusual disease clusters is an essential element in studying the spread of new infectious diseases or those intentionally released into a community, because such a cluster may be the first indication that a new disease has entered a population. And understanding the nature of heterogeneity in risk, prevalence, or incidence is an essential ingredient in determining the factors potentially affecting such heterogeneity, which can help in the design of effective control strategies. However, the majority of studies on space-time clustering center on noninfectious diseases and even those that consider infectious diseases generally stop at detection of clusters and do not consider mechanisms of spread. In addition, most studies of spatial heterogeneity of infectious diseases focus on vector-borne diseases or the effects of climate change on disease distributions. Because the focus of this review is on models for the geographic spread of infectious diseases, with emphasis on directly transmitted diseases that spread quickly across a landscape, we will provide only a brief overview of space-time clustering and spatial heterogeneity.

Several reviews of the techniques used to detect disease clustering are available (e.g., Jacquez et al., 1996a,b; Kulldorff and Nagarwalla, 1995; Kulldorff, 1998; Marshall, 1991; Waller and Jacquez, 1995; Waller and Lawson, 1995). Moore and Carpenter (1999) divide cluster detection methods into those that are concerned with point pattern data, which are represented on a map as dots or discrete locations, and those that are concerned with areal data, which are distributed continuously. The development of GIS technology, which often generates data that may be treated as spatial point patterns, has led to renewed interest in techniques used for point pattern data analysis. Traditional techniques include visual inspection of a dot map (which several researchers warned about, as it can be very misleading, especially in complex situations), statistical tests designed to detect the frequency or density of near neighbors, and tests focused on measurements of the relative distance between points. Gatrell et al. (1996) provide an overview of many of the recent methods that have been developed to analyze point pattern data. They suggest that many of the early methods for space-time clustering, including most nearest-neighbor approaches, are of limited use in epidemiological contexts, because they do not allow for spatial variation in population density, which is a critical factor influencing probability of transmission of infectious diseases. They also generally do not tie the presence of clusters to underlying risk factors (e.g., variation in water quality or personal risk behaviors) that might have generated the clustering — their purpose has often been simply to identify the presence of clusters.

Techniques for the analysis of areal data include spatial autocorrelation, Monte Carlo techniques, and calculation of specific statistics, such as Moran's I, the most commonly used statistic to estimate the level of large-scale clustering (Moore and Carpenter, 1999).[2] These analytical techniques are especially important in the study of patterns of spatial heterogeneity and help to identify how disease incidence and risk factors vary across space. In contrast to the space-time disease clustering approaches, especially in recent years studies analyzing areal data have attempted to correlate spatial heterogeneity in the distribution of risk factors with spatial heterogeneity in disease incidence and/or prevalence. Two recent studies illustrate the uses of these tech-

---

[2]Moran's I is positive when nearby areas are similar to each other and negative when they are dissimilar.

niques. Glavanakov et al. (2001) used spatial autocorrelation analysis to study the spatial character and geographic distribution of Lyme disease in New York State between 1988 and 1996. The study was done in order to understand the epizootic processes that underlay patterns of human infection, with the ultimate goal being the identification of important spatial scales for regional control. Their results showed that the regional pattern of spatial heterogeneity was consistent, even though the number of disease cases increased over time. In addition, their analysis identified three distinct disease clusters, which helped to focus control efforts in those areas most affected by the disease. Morrison et al. (1998) used GIS technology in conjunction with spatial analysis to perform a household-level analysis of dengue fever spatial patterns in a 1991-92 Puerto Rican outbreak. They found that cases appeared nearly simultaneously throughout the community, perhaps because of an insensitive surveillance system, especially early in the epidemic. Their data also suggested that mosquitoes were not very important in between-neighborhood spread, but played a significant role in within-neighborhood transmission, possibly because of natural barriers to dispersal of the *Aedes aegypti* mosquito involved in the transmission or because of low rates of mosquito survival through the pathogen incubation period. These and other results helped in the development of strategies for controlling mosquito populations in the region.

While these techniques can help to correlate disease clustering to spatially distributed risk factors, they do not prove that those risk factors are the causes of observed disease patterns. In particular, difficulties arise in the study of many human infectious diseases — transmission from human to human or from human to vector/alternate host to human is an inherently contagious process and, as such, the risk of transmission for those diseases is related not only to the occurrence of underlying risk factors, but also to the density of infectious individuals and organisms surrounding susceptible individuals. When a disease cluster is identified it can be difficult to determine whether such a cluster was due to an underlying high-risk environment or whether it was due to the presence of infectious individuals or both. If the underlying environment is not one of high risk, then observed clusters are likely to be due to the contagious process, but if this is not the case, then existing methods are not likely to be able to distinguish the causes of the observed clusters.

8.5 NEW AND POTENTIAL DIRECTIONS

At the present time much of the research on analyzing space-time patterns of infectious disease spread has depended to a large degree on retrospective analyses of past epidemics. Even forecasting models, which attempt to project disease epidemics into the future have often been performed retrospectively — by taking an older data set, using that to project the recent past, and then comparing projections with observed data to see if the projection model is reasonable. There are very few instances in the literature of studies that have attempted to project spatial patterns of epidemics into a time that is truly subsequent to the time of the study. Yet this is exactly what is needed in order to deal with newly emergent diseases or deliberately introduced infectious diseases (which are introduced in nonnatural ways) since these kinds of epidemics have not yet been seen. It is one thing to show that a model can reasonably reproduce data that have already been seen, but how do we increase our confidence in the ability of models to lead us into the unknown?

Two promising new directions within the geographic literature may prove useful in the near future. The first is the rapidly progressing development of GIS technology. At the present time the majority of GIS approaches are being used to provide better and more detailed descriptions of the degree of spatial heterogeneity in risk factors across space. Clarke et al. (1996), Gatrell and Löytönen (1998), Pfeiffer and Hugh-Jones (2002), Robinson (2000), and Rushton (1998) review the uses, limitations, and advantages of GIS approaches within epidemiology, while Boone et al. (2000), Chaput et al. (2002), Kitron and Kazmierczak (1997), McKee Jr. et al. (2000), and Moncayo et al. (2000) provide examples of specific applications. This type of knowledge would be of great value in determining realistic routes through which disease spread is likely to occur. However, the ability to effectively link the detailed and complex information contained in a GIS database with the equally complex mathematical model that would be needed to effectively model the spread of an infectious disease across space remains a major challenge in these kinds of studies.

A recent study by Tuckel et al. (2006) introduced an interesting and potentially useful intermediate step between using GIS technology to describe spatial heterogeneity and incorporating that kind of information into a dynamic model. This study, which looked at the spread of the 1918-19 influenza epidemic in Hartford, Connecticut, did not include an explicitly mathematical model, but it nonetheless considered both the temporal and spatial spread of the epidemic in a complex

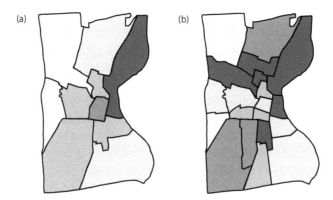

Figure 8.8 Relative rates of death and timing of deaths in different sections of
Hartford, Connecticut during the 1918-19 influenza epidemic. a) Rates
of death in each of the wards of the city. Darker colors denote higher
rates. b) Median day of death of the first five fatalities in ward subdivisions within the city. Darker colors indicate earlier spread. Adapted
from Tuckel et al. (2006), Figures 1 and 2.

and heterogeneous environment. A GIS system was developed that
included details on deaths during the epidemic, including age, date
of death, street address and city ward where the death occurred, ethnic origin, etc. This information facilitated the construction of maps
showing, for example, death rates by ward or the median date of the
first five influenza deaths in ward subdivisions (Figure 8.8). Although
the authors did not do this in their paper, it should also be possible
to make a series of maps of these types over time to generate a visual
approximation of the temporal course of the epidemic through the
city (analogous to the HIV maps shown in Figure 8.4). In this way
the GIS technology facilitates better visualization of the spatiotemporal spread of particular epidemics, but linkage of such technology
to actual dynamic models or statistical forecasting methods is needed
in order to go beyond description of past epidemics to predictions of
the course of future epidemics.

   The second new direction is the possibility of using existing infectious disease data to reconstruct mobility patterns, which would
greatly aid in the determination of pathways for disease diffusion and
help in the design of effective control strategies. At the present time
there have only been suggestions of ways to do this, with no well
worked out methods available. Disease incidence data in different
communities within larger geographic regions are routinely collected

and collated at these levels by public health authorities, however, and are much more readily available than information on contact patterns. Thus, if ways can be found to use those data to estimate the contact patterns, a major potential barrier to more widespread modeling of the geographic spread of infectious diseases might be able to be surmounted.

Three different approaches may be of use in this task, as represented by the work of Cliff and colleagues, Thomas and colleagues, and Keeling and Rohani. Cliff and Haggett (1988) suggested that spatial autocorrelation methods, which have been able to identify patterns of spatial diffusion within regions, in combination with long-term space-time series, may be of use in estimating contact patterns among communities within regions. Thomas (2001) and Smith and Thomas (2001) fit a multiregion compartmental model for HIV/AIDS transmission to data on the disease in Western and Eastern Europe. Their model assumed that the degree of contact between regions declined exponentially with distance between the regions. The model was then calibrated using recorded incidence data. Best-fit solutions were used to find estimates both of variations in the rates of mixing between regions and of the timing of epidemic spread across space.

Keeling and Rohani (2002) used a simple SIR model with coupling between two regions (represented by a simple interaction parameter) and compared it to a mechanistic model that explicitly considered the process of movement between regions. They then looked at the relationship between the coupling between regions and mechanistic mobility. Their analysis showed that in the majority of applied settings, where the return rate from interregional travel is large in comparison to the disease recovery rate, the full mechanistic model rapidly converges to the less complex coupled model and there is a simple relationship between the parameters of the two models. They also ran simulations of a stochastic or Monte Carlo version of the coupling model to compare the correlation between cases in the two model regions and the level of coupling. They showed that, for a two-group model and a few idealized multigroup models, it is possible to calculate the level of coupling and then use that information to derive the corresponding movement rates between populations. Their method thus may make it possible to reconstruct mobility patterns by observing the degree of interaction among communities, even if it is not possible to collect sufficient data on the actual mobility.

One caveat to the results of Keeling and Rohani is that they have not generalized their results beyond two regions, except for a few highly unrealistic situations. In addition, with either Keeling and

Rohani's approach or the approach of Cliff and Haggett, it will be important to assess whether different diseases will generate the same estimates of interregional mobility and contact. If that is the case, then it may be possible using one or both approaches to estimate present-day contact patterns from existing data sources. The lack of adequate information on the nature of contact patterns among groups and between individuals is one of the most significant factors hindering the widespread use of models for the geographic spread of human infectious diseases. Thus, the development of efficient techniques to approximate these contact patterns more realistically would be a major step forward on the path to more complete understanding and prediction of the geographic spread of infectious diseases.

Chapter Nine

Revisiting SARS and Looking to the Future

The vast majority of modeling studies described in the preceding pages analyzed the characteristics of past epidemics with two primary goals in mind — increasing our understanding of the specific features of the disease patterns being studied, and generating insights that could be used to help limit the spread of new outbreaks of disease. Yet except for the notable case of the 2001 U.K. foot-and-mouth epidemic, the models were not applied directly to epidemics that were ongoing at the time of the studies. And even though the foot-and-mouth disease models were developed to help with an ongoing epidemic, the disease infects domesticated animals, not humans, so the results of those models primarily inform us only about the general impact of spatial structures on the potential spread of human diseases. What have we learned from the vast amount of spatial modeling described here (including the foot-and-mouth disease models) that can be brought to bear when faced with a new epidemic of *human* disease, so that we can understand, predict, and potentially control that epidemic?

This question is no longer simply of academic interest; one major public health emergency has resulted from an infectious disease epidemic within the last few years — the 2003 SARS epidemic that we described at the beginning of this book. We return now to that epidemic and look specifically at the use of models during the epidemic and what their contributions may have been to limiting its spread.

9.1 DID MATHEMATICAL MODELING HELP TO STOP THE 2003 SARS EPIDEMIC?

A look at the headlines during the 5-month period in the winter of 2002-03 when the SARS epidemic was spreading gives a clear indication of the high level of fear that gripped the world.

CDC raises alarm over new form of pneumonia
CNN, 3/15/03

Pneumonia strain a "global threat"
CNN, 3/16/03

What next? Killer pneumonia
Time, 3/24/03

Diplomats withdrawn amid bug fears
CNN, 4/4/03

SARS: Worse than we've been told
Time, 4/8/03

Peril from the East
Time, 4/14/03

Toilet seat fears in SARS outbreak
CNN, 4/17/03

China cancels holiday over SARS
CNN, 4/21/03

... turns away students from SARS-hit regions
CNN, 5/6/03

SARS Flightmares
Time, 5/19/03

These and other headlines chronicled the distribution and impact of the epidemic and the massive public health efforts mounted worldwide to control the epidemic. Detailed studies of the early transmission and spread of the epidemic were undertaken at its outset, with clear documentation of the role of global transportation patterns in at least some cases. For example, the index patient was a doctor from Guangdong Province in China who traveled to Hong Kong for a convention. He infected at least 17 other guests and visitors at his hotel, and these secondary cases spread the disease to Vietnam, Singapore, and Toronto (Peiris et al., 2003). All affected countries and most of the rest of the world began efforts to control the outbreak as soon as its extent in initial locations became known.

Hong Kong, Spring 2003[1]

- Residents should take special care to implement personal measures such as handwashing and the use of face masks

- Patient isolation, restriction of visitors, contact tracing, and enhancement of laboratory diagnostic capacity shall be implemented

- Residents should attempt to reduce contact by limiting travel and outside social activities

- Air passengers and other travelers shall be screened for presence of infection

- The government shall keep the public informed about the epidemic through public service announcements and other actions

- Multidisciplinary investigation and response teams shall be used to enhance the effectiveness of control efforts

Singapore, Spring 2003[2]

- Contact tracing shall be implemented

- All cases and contacts of cases shall be quarantined; persons breaking quarantine shall be prosecuted

- Residents are advised to limit travel to regions experiencing SARS outbreaks

Beijing, Spring 2003[3]

- Contact tracing shall be implemented

- All cases and contacts of cases shall be quarantined

- Selected hospitals with inadequate facilities shall be closed. In return, a new hospital devoted to the treatment of SARS cases shall be built, airflow within hospitals shall be adjusted, and patients shall be aggregated in specific SARS wards

---

[1] Abdullah et al. (2003); Donnelly et al. (2003); Tsang and Lam (2003)
[2] Ooi et al. (2005)
[3] Pang et al. (2003); the new hospital was built within 7 days!

- Nonessential public facilities shall be closed

- Air passengers and other travelers shall be screened for presence of infection

Toronto, Spring 2003[4]

- Contact tracing shall be implemented

- Persons with known exposure to SARS should reduce or eliminate their exposure to others

- Residents should monitor themselves for signs of illness and seek medical care promptly if any symptoms of the disease develop

Taiwan, Spring 2003[5]

- Contact tracing shall be implemented

- All cases and contacts of cases shall be quarantined to reduce the onset-to-diagnosis time and isolate potentially infective persons more quickly from the general population

- The Ho Ping hospital shall be closed to stop hospital-based transmissions

United States, Spring 2003[6]

- A national surveillance system using a sensitive case definition that is based on all available clinical, epidemiological, and laboratory data shall be immediately implemented

- Cases shall be identified quickly and isolated and treated immediately; contact tracing shall be implemented to identify exposed contacts in an effort to limit potential spread to new areas

The examples above reflect most of the actual strategies put in place (although not necessarily the language used) in different locations to help control the epidemic. In the opinion of experts associated

---

[4]Hawryluk et al. (2004)
[5]Hsieh et al. (2004, 2005)
[6]Schrag et al. (2004)

with the SARS control efforts, contact tracing coupled with medical surveillance, isolation of cases, and quarantine of close contacts was the key to bringing the outbreak under control (Bell and WGICTS, 2004; Ooi et al., 2005; Tsang and Lam, 2003). Pang et al. (2003) and Donnelly et al. (2003) also suggested that attempts to decrease the time between illness onset and hospitalization may have been important, but Pang et al. (2003) cautioned that it was difficult to tell the degree to which these factors played a causal role.

Bell and WGICTS (2004) evaluated the specific impact of control strategies attempted by different countries. They concluded that identifying and isolating patients combined with contact tracing and treatment of contacts (if necessary) were highly effective strategies in many countries, but that quarantine and isolation also led to a number of stresses, including financial strain, psychosocial stress, and issues related to communication, compensation for lost time on the job, and workplace staffing. The strategy of attempting to monitor and/or scan people for fever was evaluated in Beijing, and was deemed not to be efficient in controlling transmission. Limitations on social activities, wearing of face masks, and increases in personal hygienic behaviors were difficult to assess because these measures were commonly implemented simultaneously with other measures. The impact of travel advisories was also difficult to assess because there were additional sources of information available to travelers. Assessment of measures designed to screen travelers at international borders had many associated problems, including, for example, difficulties separating entry from exit screening in the recorded data, determining whether travelers entered from affected countries, and isolating data dating to the epidemic itself from a transportation data set collated over a longer period of time. Transmission on commercial aircraft was clearly documented (Breugelmans et al., 2004), but determining actual transmission risks from the available data was very difficult. Bell and WGICTS (2004) concluded that traditional public health interventions were most important in containing the spread of the epidemic, but that such methods may not work as well for more readily transmissible infections. They also cautioned that political and economic factors and the social consequences of control policies must be considered at all times.

What role, if any, did mathematical modeling play in the implementation, duration of use, or assessment of any of these strategies? In order to answer this question, it is necessary to take a look at the specific models that were brought into play, at the kinds of insights they provided, and at the likelihood that those insights were made available to those health authorities who were in a position to make use of them.

Models published while the epidemic was in progress or shortly thereafter represent the work of individuals who were most likely in a position to influence public health authorities, but only a small number of such models were published (e.g., Chau and Yip, 2003; Chowell et al., 2003; Lipsitch et al., 2003; Lloyd-Smith et al., 2003; Riley et al., 2003). These models clearly had the potential to influence public health authorities, but it is difficult to know how much actual communication the modelers might have had with the authorities. It is also difficult to determine whether modelers who published their work slightly later were in communication with the authorities prior to the publication of their work. Examples of the latter work include Chowell et al. (2004), Gumel et al. (2004), Hufnagel et al. (2004), Meyers et al. (2005), Wallinga and Teunis (2004), and Webb et al. (2004). In addition to publication after the end of the epidemic, however, these later models generally seem to be assessing the epidemic after the fact rather than while it was in progress.

The first two papers presenting models for the spread of SARS were those of Lipsitch et al. (2003) and Riley et al. (2003), which were published online simultaneously on 23 May 2003 in the journal *Science*, along with a commentary on the two papers by Dye and Gay (2003). Lipsitch et al. (2003) used a combination of simple deterministic modeling and stochastic modeling to estimate the infectiousness of the SARS virus, to determine how likely an outbreak would be if the virus were introduced into a fully susceptible population, and to assess, at least in a preliminary fashion, the efficacy of different control strategies. Using their model, they derived an approximate estimate of the basic reproductive number, R_0, which ranged from 2.2 to 3.6. Since this range of values is lower than estimates for most other respiratory diseases, Lipsitch et al. (2003) suggested that SARS would be easier to control than the average respiratory infection, but that it could still spread if unchecked. In addition, they pointed out that although at the time of their study there appeared to be little evidence for transmission by asymptomatic cases, if that became significant, then it would make the epidemic much harder to control.

Lipsitch et al. (2003) also looked at two major control strategies — isolation of symptomatic cases and close observation and quarantine of close contacts of cases. Their analyses led them to conclude that a combination of control measures, including shortening the time from the onset of symptoms to isolation of cases and implementing effective contact tracing and quarantine of exposed persons, could help to control the spread of the epidemic.

Riley et al. (2003) used a stochastic metapopulation compartmental model and derived conclusions similar to those of Lipsitch et al. (2003). They generated an estimate for R_0 of 2.7, although as Dye and Gay (2003) point out, in determining this estimate they did not include superspreaders, which were a known feature of this epidemic. Ignoring obvious heterogeneity in transmission related to the presence of superspreaders emphasizes low-transmission events and ignores the potential for additional localized outbreaks to be generated by a small number of individuals who transmit to high numbers of individuals (Dye and Gay, 2003).

Besides their similar estimate of R_0, Riley et al. (2003) came to the same general conclusions as Lipsitch et al. (2003) about which control strategies might be effective; namely, that isolation of cases combined with contact tracing and quarantining of contacts were appropriate and effective strategies. One difference in their results, however, was that they concluded that such strategies *already had been* effective, at least in Hong Kong, while Lipsitch et al. (2003) concluded only that they *could* be effective (Dye and Gay, 2003). One factor considered by Riley et al. (2003) but not Lipsitch et al. (2003) was the effect of between-district contact patterns. As a result of this analysis, Riley et al. (2003) concluded that restricting movement might have a substantial impact, especially if other strategies, such as reducing the time from symptom onset to hospitalization, could not be implemented effectively.

Three other papers, Chau and Yip (2003), Chowell et al. (2003), and Lloyd-Smith et al. (2003), presented work that appeared to be completed while the epidemic was still in progress. Chau and Yip (2003) used a statistical technique, back projection, to estimate the infection curve and assess the effectiveness of interventions in Hong Kong. Like Lipsitch et al. (2003) and Riley et al. (2003), they suggested that quarantining cases and close contacts of those cases were key factors in stemming the spread of the epidemic (which was nearly over at the time they completed their study). Chowell et al. (2003) used a deterministic compartmental model to estimate epidemiological parameters from Toronto, Hong Kong, and Singapore. Their results suggested that rapid diagnosis and quick isolation of cases could have a major impact on the spread of the disease. Lloyd-Smith et al. (2003) used a stochastic model to focus on the spread of the disease within a community and its associated hospital, and they also paid special attention to modeling realistic incubation and symptomatic periods since these are less variable in different epidemics than are mixing and transmission patterns. Their results suggested that hospital-based containment measures would be most effective in controlling disease spread, especially in the case of inadequate screening of health care workers, and that mechanisms to control contact between health care workers and the general community would be essential elements of effective control strategies.

In general, most of these early SARS modeling efforts focused on estimating R_0, as well as evaluating potential control strategies. Estimates of R_0 consistently fell around 3, suggesting a disease that was moderately infectious. Other parameters besides R_0 that were found to be important in one or more of these early models were the proportion of transmissions occurring before symptoms became apparent, the variance in the number of secondary cases produced per infected individual, and heterogeneity in the number of contacts. Model analyses also consistently concluded that the best strategies to use in minimizing epidemic spread were the traditional epidemiological strategies of isolation of cases, contact tracing, and quarantining of exposed individuals. (For an excellent critique of these models and a discussion of the kinds of conclusions that are best derived through the use of mathematical models, see Bauch et al. (2005).)

What were the contributions of models that appeared after the epidemic subsided? The majority of these studies reinforced the results of the earlier models. For example, Chowell et al. (2004) concluded that multiple control methods were necessary. Gumel et al. (2004) concluded that isolation of patients was critical, and Gumel et al. (2004) and Webb et al. (2004) suggested that quarantine would be most effective when combined with isolation of cases. Other models indicated that a quick and focused reaction was essential to limit global spread (Hufnagel et al., 2004) and general spread (Wallinga and Teunis, 2004) of the epidemic. Meyers et al. (2005) used an individual, network-based simulation to demonstrate that two epidemics with the same R_0 could nonetheless generate very different epidemics due to the nature of connections linking individuals within the affected populations. They thus pointed out the critical importance of the contact structure of a population in determining patterns of epidemic spread and suggested that the total estimated number of contacts during the infectious period is at least as important a parameter as the number of new infections per case (as estimated by R_0).

So, when all is said and done, did mathematical models really help to control the spread of the SARS epidemic? In our opinion, the answer to this question is a qualified "yes." Mathematical models confirmed the importance of traditional strategies used to contain infectious disease epidemics, but those strategies were the first choice of epidemiologists in any case. More importantly, however, because SARS was a new disease, no one knew how fast it was capable of spreading, where it might spread, and who was at greatest risk for the disease. Mathematical models were used to compute estimates of critical parameters, such as R_0, that provided initial ideas of the potential seriousness of the problem, and they were fine-tuned throughout the epidemic to help assess progress in attempts to control it. They were used to explore unknown territory in relation to the disease, such as the consequences of potentially inadequate estimation of the extent of asymptomatic transmission and other fundamental characteristics of infectious disease transmission systems.

Mathematical models thus provided a new tool to bring into play during a major public health emergency, and, although attributes of the SARS virus, such as its relatively low infectiousness and limited degree of transmission by infectious persons when asymptomatic, may have allowed the epidemic to be controlled solely through traditional public health approaches, the unusual biology of the virus compared to other respiratory viruses made the success of those traditional methods much more likely. We may not be so lucky with the next new virus, and may well be glad that we are developing so many new tools with which to analyze and assess potential control strategies.

9.2 MODELING THE GEOGRAPHIC SPREAD OF PAST, PRESENT, AND FUTURE INFECTIOUS DISEASE EPIDEMICS: LESSONS AND ADVICE

The previous chapters have presented an extensive overview of the kinds of models and techniques that have been used to study the geographic spread of infectious diseases and they have illustrated how these techniques have been applied to real-world epidemics. In the last part of this final chapter we summarize and reinforce what we think are the most important concepts related to spatial modeling and provide some guidelines to follow in taking on the challenge of developing a new model and/or applying such a model to the spread across time and space of a human infectious disease epidemic.

9.2.1 The major issues addressed by spatial models

Nonspatial models have provided important insights and guidance in determining effective community-wide control policies and strategies, but as a consequence of a growing awareness of the ways modern rates of travel are leading to the development of a truly global community, epidemiologists have expanded their sights to consider more extensive strategies for between-community control in addition to the traditional within-community approaches. In these situations it is essential to use spatial models to assess the risks of epidemic spread from one community to others and to aid in developing efficient and effective means for stemming such epidemics. As our examples in the previous pages have shown, the most important issues that have been addressed by spatial models in the present literature include

1) elucidating broad-scale patterns of spread across space, including predictions of where outbreaks are likely to spread and when they will reach different communities,

2) predicting the rate of advance of epidemic waves following introduction,

3) developing an understanding of how and why diseases persist over time and space and the role of different factors in maintaining persistence or promoting extinction at different geographic scales,

4) exploring how different contact structures between communities and individuals promote or inhibit the spread of a disease across time and space,

5) determining the degree of synchronization of epidemics in different communities within a region and the importance of that synchronization for maintaining the prevalence of a disease or facilitating extinction within the region,

6) predicting the periodicity of disease prevalence patterns and identifying the role of factors that influence that periodicity, and

7) determining reasonable control strategies and evaluating their effectiveness in containing an outbreak of an infectious disease so that it does not spread outside of the initial local region, and using model insights to help direct those control strategies to where they might do the most good.

Much is now known in relation to some of these issues, while others are less certain. For example, as Chapter 5 showed, mathematical epidemiologists have developed models that are fairly successful in explaining the persistence, periodicity, and synchrony of measles epidemics, although there are still significant questions that have not been completely answered. Predicting where and when a new epidemic will spread is still a wide open question. We do not have a particularly good understanding of how, why, and especially when past epidemics may spread from an index community to other communities across a landscape and so our ability to gauge this for epidemics yet to come is relatively limited. A big part of the reason for this is that we still don't know very much about the contact patterns that link different individuals and communities together. A lot of attention, both practical and theoretical, is being devoted to this issue, but much work remains. Much work is also needed on assessing the appropriateness and effectiveness of different control strategies and, perhaps more importantly, on figuring out how models can best be used to improve traditional strategies. As the experiences during both the 2001 U.K. foot-and-mouth disease epidemic and the 2003 SARS epidemic clearly showed, traditional and standard epidemiological practices were at least as effective as mathematical modeling efforts (which to a greater or lesser degree simply validated those practices). Mathematical models are an important new tool, but additional work is needed both to determine their optimal role in the development of control strategies and to convince public health authorities that they have much to offer.

9.2.2 A strategy for taking on the challenge of spatial modeling

So how does one begin to tackle the task of spatial modeling? In this book we have discussed many concepts and issues that should be kept in mind when developing and analyzing mathematical models. We review many of those ideas here, but in the context of the process involved in actually devising and implementing a model of the geographic spread of an infectious disease.

Before attempting to develop an actual mathematical or computer model for the geographic spread of an infectious disease, it is helpful to ask several basic questions. In many cases, the process of deriving answers to these questions will suggest the type of modeling approach to use and the initial steps to take in deriving the model. Figure 9.1 highlights the issues discussed below and how they relate to the three major modeling approaches — population-based mathematical models, individual-based mathematical models, and computer simulation (including Monte Carlo simulation, agent-based models, and other simulation techniques).

Question 1. What is the overall purpose of the model and the specific questions to be addressed?

This question is probably the most important question of all (hence its prominent position at the head of the line). Models that are intended primarily to advance our theoretical understanding of the role of space will often and probably should be somewhat different from those that are intended for practical use in predicting and controlling the spread of an epidemic. In particular, mathematical approaches are better suited for theory building than are computer simulations, although the latter can be and often are developed in conjunction with mathematical approaches. Specific questions addressed by mathematical approaches include questions about the long-term time dynamics of a model, the existence of equilibria and the stability of those equilibria, the conditions under which a disease will either go extinct or remain endemic in a population, and similar kinds of questions.

Mathematical approaches usually lead to models that are more general and applicable to a wide variety of situations, and their analysis results in greater understanding of the impact different assumptions may have on patterns of disease spread. This kind of knowledge is invaluable in interpreting the results from either mathematical models that have been designed for a particular practical purpose or computer simulations focused on practical questions. Although some theoretical analyses are of use in practical situations (e.g., determining conditions for extinction), theoretical models are likely to contain simplifications that make them less realistic and applicable to the particular problem being addressed. Conversely, models developed to address particular practical problems may not be amenable to mathematical or other theoretical analyses and their applicability to more general questions may be limited.

With reference to the different kinds of models discussed in this book, the simpler, population-based spatial models (spatially continuous and some of the metapopulation models) are more amenable to general mathematical analyses than are more complex models, but they are also less realistic. Individual-based models are usually the most realistic, but their underlying mathematical structure may not be explicit, which limits their ability to be analyzed mathematically. Some individual-based models do have an explicit mathematical structure, but even in those cases, the structure may not be conducive to extensive mathematical analyses. In addition, as a group, deterministic models are generally less complex and more able to be analyzed mathematically than stochastic models, but deterministic models can-

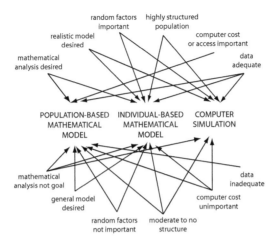

Figure 9.1 Suggested model types to use when dealing with different modeling issues. Arrows lead to a model type that ought to be considered when a particular situation is of importance for a project.

not effectively capture the inherent randomness of real epidemic situations. This randomness can be included in stochastic models at either the individual or population level, but is perhaps most easily incorporated at the individual level. However, because of the limited degree of mathematical analysis possible with most individual-based models and because they often have a complex and specific model structure, the results of such models may not be generalizable to situations they were not designed to address.

If the primary purpose of a model is to expand our theoretical understanding of how epidemics spread across space and time, then ensuring that the model is amenable to mathematical analysis will be a primary concern. If the primary purpose is to answer a specific practical question, however, then the necessary assumptions needed to guarantee that a model is amenable to significant mathematical analysis may well compromise the ability of that model to effectively address the question. Of course, for many questions both mathematical and practical approaches are useful, and the successful integration of these two approaches can lead to additional advances above and beyond each approach alone. When all is said and done, the questions to be addressed, the biology of the disease being modeled, and the available data with which to validate models should be the prime factors motivating the choice of modeling approach.

Question 2. What kind of population will be modeled?

The characteristics of the population to be modeled can also help to dictate the best modeling approach to use, especially in a spatial framework where complexity can build up rapidly. The majority of spatial models that have provided useful and practical insights into the geographic spread of actual epidemics have used either a metapopulation approach or an individual-based structure. Deciding between these two strategies depends in large part on the size of the population being modeled, the geographic scale, the amount of information on the contact networks both available and needed to address the specific questions of interest, and the questions themselves.

In general, if the population of interest is very small, then stochastic effects can become extremely important, and so the modeling approach should allow the incorporation of such effects. The methods underlying most metapopulation and other population-based models usually assume that populations are large and they usually do not incorporate much or any stochasticity. Although initial analyses of such models for smaller populations can be a good first step, individual-based models are generally more appropriate and will provide more realistic answers to questions of interest. Of course, if the questions of interest are at the level of the entire population rather than at the individual level, then it is best to use both population- and individual-based approaches, even for small populations, since the population-based models are amenable to theoretical analyses that provide a better base for the interpretation of results from the individual-based approaches.

Depending on the questions of interest, stochastic effects can be an important consideration. This is especially the case if one wants to study the early stages of an epidemic when the number of infectious individuals is small. In that situation, even if the overall population is huge, the probability of extinction of an epidemic within a community is high. Spatial models that allow for repeated reintroductions of a disease into communities within a larger region suggest that the spatial structure and interconnectedness among communities present in real populations can offset the trend for stochastic effects to cause local extinction and enhance the persistence of a disease at the regional level. On the other hand, stochasticity prevents one from making extremely detailed predictions of when and where an outbreak will occur — a desired, but likely unattainable outcome of mathematical modeling activities.

If populations are large and one is interested in what happens once an epidemic takes hold, then a population-based approach may be reasonable. The computational costs in both time and money are generally much less for such approaches, and because the models tend to be simpler in structure, they are more likely to be amenable to mathematical analyses. Thus, much can be learned relatively quickly and inexpensively about the general behavior of the system being modeled.

Several other factors can influence the choice of whether to use a population-based or individual-based model, including the type of geographic structure present in the population being considered, the geographic scale at which one wants to observe epidemic behavior, and the composition of the study population. The impact of these factors is closely tied to the issue of population size. The greater the level of geographic structuring, the smaller the individual subpopulations tend to be, and so the greater the need to seriously consider individual-based approaches. Greater levels of geographic structuring imply smaller geographic scales (e.g., consideration of individual towns rather than districts, or consideration of neighborhoods rather than cities as a whole). The population composition can also lead to smaller-scale structures, as, for example, when a population is subdivided into different age classes. Population-level models can be and have been developed to describe many of these situations, but they can quickly become so complex in structure that they lose the advantages generally associated with the simpler population-based approaches.

The structure of contacts within and among groups is also an essential factor to consider when deciding on a modeling approach, especially in a spatial context. As has been repeatedly emphasized, the patterns of contact in human populations are not well understood at almost all levels. A model is only as good as the data that underlie it (more on this below), and although it might be attractive to consider a highly subdivided population, if the information on rates of contact between groups is inadequate then the model will not be able to answer the questions at a level of confidence that would be desirable. For example, it might be really interesting to study how measles spreads among different ethnic enclaves in a city, but if one knows little about how individuals from different enclaves come into contact with one another and bases estimates of those patterns totally on assumptions (which may well be unfounded if there are no data to anchor them), then the model will not be able to generate realistic results.

Again, the nature of the specific questions to be addressed will help to make the choice of model clearer. Many of the influenza models described in Chapter 3 effectively used metapopulation or similar models, since the questions of interest were to identify global or regional patterns of spread of the disease. At such scales, detailed model structures (and the data required for them) are not really needed, since observed patterns at such a level are not very detailed themselves. On the other hand, if detailed understanding of specific patterns of localized spread are desired and/or if stochasticity is an important consideration, then individual-based models are preferred. In the best of all possible worlds, of course, both population- and individual-based models will be used to study the same scenario, since they may well give different kinds of information that can be combined to produce even more effective outcomes.

Question 3. What are the biological and epidemiological characteristics of the disease?

In order to effectively model the transmission of any infectious disease, it is essential to know as much as possible about the biological and epidemiological characteristics of the disease. This is especially important for practical models, but it is also important for theoretical models since a model that is not well grounded in reality will be less likely to generate analytical results that are of relevance to real-world problems.

At the minimum, the course of infection in an individual needs to be known so that the relevant disease statuses (susceptible, exposed, infectious, etc.) can be modeled. Assumptions also need to be made about the different stages of infection. Assumptions of the simplest models include a constant rate of transmission and recovery, and in many cases these assumptions are reasonable as a first approximation. There are many interesting questions, however, for which these assumptions are not reasonable. For example, in reality the length of time different individuals are infectious is probably quite variable as a consequence of factors such as differential underlying health status and use of prophylactic measures. Consequently, a modeler may want to allow for a variable rate of infection or recovery.

In addition to these kinds of issues, which are relevant to all epidemic models, spatial models have the additional problem of multiple subpopulations. Most models assume that the underlying disease biology and epidemiology is the same for all subpopulations, but this need not be the case. For example, if one is modeling the spread of a waterborne disease among different communities, the risks of transmission may vary dramatically due to varying levels of sanitary facilities. In such a case, allowing transmission risks to vary in the model may be necessary in order to develop an adequate model. It is important to remember, however, that relaxing assumptions about homogeneity across groups increases the need for detailed within-group data, a factor that may well offset any benefits gained by incorporating more realistic assumptions.

Question 4. What kinds of data are available?

Data issues are a pressing matter, especially for models of a practical nature, where they may be a serious roadblock to progress. The success of spatial models in aiding in the development of effective strategies to control the spread of epidemics and minimize their impact on the affected human populations has hinged on the existence of suitable and adequate data sets with which to estimate model parameters. Data availability and quality are probably the weakest links in the chain of events leading from model development to effective control policies, however, especially in a geographic framework. Spatial epidemic models need both epidemic data collected in different communities within a region and data on the patterns of interaction and mobility that link the communities together. Network models require information on both the individuals in the population and the contacts those individuals have with others. It is extremely rare for all the necessary types of data to be available for the same epidemic. Much attention is being devoted to finding better ways to approximate the needed data using more readily available information. This work is still limited in its practical uses, however, pointing to the serious need for spatially detailed information on both disease and contact rates and patterns.

It is important to become familiar with potential data sources before settling on a model structure. Particularly for geographic and network models, the task of collecting the necessary data is time-consuming, expensive, and almost certainly beyond the capabilities of most modelers. Even if some data of the right type are available, they may be of poor quality, they may be lacking in sufficient detail, the reporting intervals may be too long for the questions being considered, or the data may be aggregated across groups that do not relate well to the purpose of the desired model. Recall the Russian flu simulations of Baroyan and colleagues described in Chapter 3. Although the simulations could be run for all of the cities in the study, the epidemiological data in most localities were collected only monthly, a period of time that was too long to be able to see much of the detail of a short-lived flu epidemic. As another example, a modeler may like to consider the spread of a disease through a group of preschool children, but upon checking into potential data sources, he or she may find that the most important data are aggregated into 5-year age groups (a common way to present demographic data), a level of aggregation that lumps essentially all of the important heterogeneity into one homogeneous group. These kinds of constraints need to be kept in mind when deciding on the kind of model to use, so that a model structure that is appropriate for the question to be studied will also have adequate data available with which to estimate the essential parameters.

The detailed geographic patterns of an epidemic can be neither replicated nor predicted exactly, partly because of the inherently stochastic nature of real epidemics and partly because of a lack of adequate spatial data. But in spite of this inherent limitation, models based on the highest quality of data can provide better insights than logically based impressions and conclusions. Throughout the book we have attempted to highlight those studies we think are exemplary and have used them to illustrate both the advantages and disadvantages of using mathematical modeling approaches to predict patterns of epidemic spread and adequate methods of control. Our review of this body of research leads us to a few cautions and final thoughts about the use of these spatial modeling approaches, with which we end our book.

9.2.3 Cautions and concluding thoughts

The increasing globalization of the world and the possibility that pathogens may be released deliberately have led to significant changes in the risk of rapid geographic spread of infectious diseases. The deliberate release of pathogens is likely to result in patterns of spread that are qualitatively different from natural epidemics because they are more likely to enter a population from multiple sources simultaneously in situations designed to maximize the rate of spread through a population, and the globalization of the world guarantees that both naturally occurring and deliberately released pathogens have the potential to spread quickly to all corners of the Earth. Existing epidemiological data are derived from natural epidemics that occurred in the past; thus, traditional control strategies derived from statistical analyses of these data may not be applicable to either newly evolving pathogens or those introduced through bioterrorism. Mathematical models are an ideal method to use in determining critical parameter estimates and in exploring the potential patterns of spread of new diseases, because as long as enough data are available to make reasonable assumptions about unknowns, the techniques of mathematical modeling are particularly well-suited to situations where there is little prior experience and existing data.

While exceedingly valuable in understanding the spread of infectious diseases, mathematical models have their limitations and must not be used indiscriminately. Stochasticity prevents one from making extremely detailed predictions of when and where an outbreak will occur — usually only statistical assessments (e.g., averages and uncertainties) are possible. Furthermore, in spatial settings, incidence patterns may be highly sensitive to a small number of long-range transmission events, which are likely to be extremely difficult to predict. Model predictions can also be highly dependent on model assumptions in some cases (for example, predicted rates of spread are significantly influenced by how the infectious period is modeled).

There is a great need for spatial epidemic models. Nonspatial models are suitable for predicting who gets infected, and when and why they get infected within a single population, but geographic models are needed to address questions of where a disease will spread, the timing of spread to different communities, and the reasons for those patterns of spread. Unfortunately, only a small number of spatial models have addressed practical issues using high-quality data sources to estimate model parameters.

A variety of approaches are needed to address questions of interest in the spatial spread of infectious diseases. One model or type of model will not be appropriate for all potential diseases and questions. Furthermore, stronger conclusions are possible when the results of a variety of approaches addressing similar questions are compared. The choice of approach must be linked to 1) the biology of the disease being modeled, 2) the questions needed to be answered with a model, and 3) the nature of existing data. The most realistic models may not be the most useful if, as is often the case, adequate data to estimate model parameters are not available. In addition, in some cases simpler models may provide results that are adequate for the question at hand, but decisions to use the simpler models must be made carefully and after serious evaluation of the potential impact of their assumptions on patterns of disease spread.

Models without spatial structure (i.e., homogeneously mixing models) generally result in worst-case scenarios. Thus, such models will be conservative. Policies derived from them may be acceptable for short-term or crisis decisions, but their use may be less reasonable in larger-scale situations, where costs as well as benefits must be taken into account. For example, they may be more expensive than necessary or they may be overly disruptive or risky.

A lot of effort is spent on calculating R_0 and other simple quantities derived from models because they provide a quick way to get some indication of the potential for significant disease transmission. Caution must be exercised in basing policy solely on such calculations, however, because they are model dependent and may be misleading if the underlying model is inadequate. For example, the calculated R_0 for measles is known to be well above one at the population level, which would suggest disease persistence, but more sophisticated models have clearly shown that stochastic effects can lead to local nonpersistence (although spatial effects can counteract this local extinction tendency). It is also important to realize that parameter estimates derived from a given population context (e.g., a hospital outbreak) may not apply to another (e.g., a city-level outbreak).

One should be wary of model predictions that fit too well, particularly when the data underlying the model are inadequate or of uncertain quality. Furthermore, model fits should be assessed in light of the number of free parameters. Models can fit for the wrong reasons — good fits don't necessarily imply that one has captured the underlying mechanisms.

GIS technology is generating large data sets that may be of use in studies of the spatial spread of infectious diseases. However, much work still needs to be done on developing ways to place the extensive data sets produced by the GIS technology within a dynamic framework that can predict present and future patterns of disease spread across space and time. Without the development of effective ways to link GIS data and dynamic models, the advantages of the sophisticated technology will continue to be limited to descriptive studies of spatial heterogeneity.

Mathematical and computer models for the geographic spread of infectious diseases are rapidly becoming an important component of programs designed to better predict and control outbreaks of infectious diseases at the local, regional, national, and global scales. In order to ensure that such models reach their potential in aiding these efforts, model development and analysis must proceed through multidisciplinary collaborations among mathematicians, statisticians, biologists, epidemiologists, social scientists, and others with expertise in infectious disease studies. It is only through such groups that the models will have appropriate levels of mathematical detail, that they capture the essential elements of the biology of host, pathogen, and other organisms involved in the disease life cycle, and that they retain an appreciation for the complexities of human activities, needs, and desires and how these may influence and be affected by disease outbreaks. The studies described in this book represent only the first steps towards bringing the powerful new techniques of mathematical modeling together with traditional approaches to public health. Such a union can only increase our success in dealing with future epidemics.

·

Bibliography

Abdullah, A. S. M., Tomlinson, B., Cockram, C. S., and Thomas, G. N. (2003). Lessons from the severe acute respiratory syndrome outbreak in Hong Kong. *Emerging Infectious Diseases*, 9(9):1042–1045.

Ackerman, E., Elveback, L., and Fox, J. P. (1984). *Simulation of Infectious Disease Epidemics*. Charles C. Thomas, Springfield, IL.

Adesina, H. O. (1984). Identification of the cholera diffusion process in Ibadan, 1971. *Social Science and Medicine*, 18(5):429–440.

Adler, F. R. (1992). The effects of averaging on the basic reproduction ratio. *Mathematical Biosciences*, 111(1):89–98.

Aguirre, A. and Gonzalez, E. (1992). The feasibility of forecasting influenza epidemics in Cuba. *Memorias do Instituto Oswaldo Cruz*, 87(3):429–432.

Albert, R., Jeong, H., and Barabási, A. L. (2000). Error and attack tolerance of complex networks. *Nature*, 406:378–382.

Anderson, D. and Watson, R. (1980). On the spread of a disease with gamma distributed latent and infectious periods. *Biometrika*, 67:191–198.

Anderson, R. M. (1982). Transmission dynamics and control of infectious disease agents. In Anderson, R. M. and May, R. M., editors, *Population Biology of Infectious Diseases*, pages 149–176. Springer-Verlag, New York.

Anderson, R. M., Grenfell, B. T., and May, R. M. (1984). Oscillatory fluctuations in the incidence of infectious disease and the impact of vaccination: Time series analysis. *Journal of Hygiene–Cambridge*, 93(3):587–608.

Anderson, R. M., Jackson, H. C., May, R. M., and Smith, A. M. (1981). Population dynamics of fox rabies in Europe. *Nature*, 289(5800):765–771.

Anderson, R. M. and May, R. M. (1991). *Infectious Diseases of Humans: Dynamics and Control*. Oxford University Press, Oxford.

Anderson, R. M., May, R. M., and McLean, A. R. (1988). Possible demographic consequences of AIDS in developing countries. *Nature*, 332(6161):228–234.

Anderson, R. M., Medley, G. F., May, R. M., and Johnson, A. M. (1986). A preliminary study of the transmission dynamics of the human immunodeficiency virus (HIV), the causative agent of AIDS. *IMA Journal of Mathematics Applied in Medicine and Biology*, 3(4):229–263.

Anderson, R. M., Ng, T. W., Boily, M. C., and May, R. M. (1989). The influence of different sexual-contact patterns between age classes on the predicted demographic impact of AIDS in developing countries. *Annals of the New York Academy of Science*, 569:240–274.

Andersson, H. (1997). Epidemics in a population with social structures. *Mathematical Biosciences*, 140:79–84.

Andersson, H. (1998). Limit theorems for a random graph epidemic model. *Annals of Applied Probability*, 8:1331–1349.

Andersson, H. and Britton, T. (2000a). *Stochastic Epidemic Models and Their Analysis*. Springer-Verlag, New York.

Andersson, H. and Britton, T. (2000b). Stochastic epidemics in dynamic populations: Quasi-stationarity and extinction. *Journal of Mathematical Biology*, 41(6):559–580.

Andreasen, V. and Christiansen, F. B. (1989). Persistence of an infectious disease in a subdivided population. *Mathematical Biosciences*, 96:239–253.

Angulo, J. J., Haggett, P., Megale, P., and Pederneiras, A. A. (1977). Variola minor in Braganca Paulista county, 1956: A trend-surface analysis. *American Journal of Epidemiology*, 105(3):272–278.

Antonovics, J., Iwasa, Y., and Hassell, M. P. (1995). A generalized model of parasitoid, venereal, and vector-based transmission processes. *American Naturalist*, 145:661–675.

Aparicio, J. P. and Solari, H. G. (2001a). Population dynamics: Poisson approximation and its relation to the Langevin process. *Physical Review Letters*, 86(18):4183–4186.

Aparicio, J. P. and Solari, H. G. (2001b). Sustained oscillations in stochastic systems. *Mathematical Biosciences*, 169(1):15–25.

Arino, J., Davis, J. R., Hartley, D., Jordan, R., Miller, J. M., and van den Driessche, P. (2005). A multi-species epidemic model with spatial dynamics. *Mathematical Medicine and Biology*, 22:129–142.

Arino, J. and van den Driessche, P. (2003). A multi-city epidemic model. *Mathematical Population Studies*, 10(3):175–193.

Aron, J. L. and May, R. M. (1982). The population dynamics of
malaria. In Anderson, R. M., editor, *Population Dynamics of Infectious Diseases: Theory and Applications*, pages 139–179. Chapman
and Hall, London.

Assunção, R. M., Reis, I. A., and Oliveira, C. D. (2001). Diffusion
and prediction of Leishmaniasis in a large metropolitan area in
Brazil with a Bayesian space-time model. *Statistics in Medicine*,
20(15):2319–2335.

Bailey, N. T. J. (1964). Some stochastic models for small epidemics in
large populations. *Journal of the Royal Statistical Society, Series
C, Applied Statistics*, 13:9–19.

Bailey, N. T. J. (1975). *The Mathematical Theory of Infectious Diseases and Its Applications*. Hafner, New York.

Ball, F. and Neal, P. (2008). Network epidemic models with two levels
of mixing. *Mathematical Biosciences*, 212:69–87.

Ball, F. G. (1985). Spatial models for the spread and control of rabies
incorporating group size. In Bacon, P., editor, *Population Dynamics
of Rabies in Wildlife*, pages 197–221. Academic Press, London.

Ball, F. G. (1991). Dynamic population epidemic models. *Mathematical Biosciences*, 107(2):299–324.

Ball, F. G. (1995). Coupling methods in epidemic theory. In Mollison,
D., editor, *Epidemic Models: Their Structure and Relation to Data*,
pages 34–52. Cambridge University Press, Cambridge.

Ball, F. G., Mollison, D., and Scalia-Tomba, G. (1997). Epidemics
with two levels of mixing. *Annals of Applied Probability*, 7:46–89.

Barabási, A. L. (2003). *Linked: How Everything Is Connected to
Everything Else and What It Means for Business, Science, and Everyday Life*. Plume, New York.

Barabási, A. L. and Albert, R. (1999). Emergence of scaling in random
networks. *Science*, 286(5439):509–512.

Barbour, A. and Mollison, D. (1990). Epidemics and random graphs.
In Gabriel, J.-P., Lefévre, C., and Picard, P., editors, *Stochastic
Processes in Epidemic Theory*, Lecture Notes in Biomathematics
86, pages 86–89. Springer-Verlag, New York.

Barbour, A. D. (1978). Macdonald's model and the transmission of
bilharzia. *Transactions of the Royal Society of Tropical Medicine
and Hygiene*, 72(1):6–15.

Baroyan, O. V., Basilevsky, U. V., Ermakov, V. V., Frank, K. D.,
Rvachev, L. A., and Shashkov, V. A. (1970). Computer modelling
of influenza epidemics for large-scale systems of cities and territo-

ries. Working paper for WHO Symposium on Quantitative Epidemiology.

Baroyan, O. V., Genchikov, L. A., Rvachev, L. A., and Schaschkov, V. A. (1969). An attempt at large-scale influenza modelling by means of a computer. *Bulletin of the International Epidemiological Association*, 18:22–31.

Baroyan, O. V. and Rvachev, L. A. (1967). Deterministic models of epidemics for a territory with a transport network. *Kibernetika (Cybernetics)*, 3:67–74.

Baroyan, O. V. and Rvachev, L. A. (1978). Prediction of influenza epidemics in the USSR. (in Russian). *Voprosy Virusologii*, 2:131–137.

Baroyan, O. V., Rvachev, L. A., Basilevsky, U. V., Ermakov, V. V., Frank, K. D., Rvachev, M. A., and Shashkov, V. A. (1971). Computer modelling of influenza epidemics for the whole country (USSR). *Advances in Applied Probability*, 3:224–226.

Baroyan, O. V., Rvachev, L. A., Frank, K., and et al. (1978). Model of influenza epidemics spread through the territory of Bulgaria and its significance. (in Bulgarian). *Journal of Epidemiology, Microbiology, and Infectious Diseases (Sofia)*, 3:168–173.

Bartlett, M. S. (1954). Processus stochastiques ponctuels. *Annales de l'Institut Henri Poincare*, 14:35.

Bartlett, M. S. (1956). Deterministic and stochastic models for recurrent epidemics. *Proceedings of the 3rd Berkeley Symposium on Mathematics, Statistics, and Probability*, 4:81–109.

Bartlett, M. S. (1957). Measles periodicity and community size. *Journal of the Royal Statistical Society, Series A, Statistics in Society*, 120:48–70.

Bartlett, M. S. (1960a). The critical community size for measles in the United States. *Journal of the Royal Statistical Society, Series A, Statistics in Society*, 123:37–44.

Bartlett, M. S. (1960b). *Stochastic Population Models in Ecology and Epidemiology*. Methuen, London.

Bartlett, M. S. (1964). The relevance of stochastic models for large-scale epidemic phenomena. *Journal of the Royal Statistical Society, Series C, Applied Statistics*, 13:2–8.

Bates, T. W., Thurmond, M. C., and Carpenter, T. E. (2003a). Description of an epidemic simulation model for use in evaluating strategies to control an outbreak of foot-and-mouth disease. *American Journal of Veterinary Research*, 64(2):195–204.

Bates, T. W., Thurmond, M. C., and Carpenter, T. E. (2003b). Epidemiologic information for modeling foot-and-mouth disease. In Banks, H. T. and Castillo-Chavez, C., editors, *Bioterrorism: Mathematical Modeling Applications in Homeland Security*, pages 107–127. Society for Industrial and Applied Mathematics, Philadelphia.

Bates, T. W., Thurmond, M. C., and Carpenter, T. E. (2003c). Results of epidemic simulation modeling to evaluate strategies to control an outbreak of foot-and-mouth disease. *American Journal of Veterinary Research*, 64(2):205–210.

Bauch, C. (2002). A versatile ODE approximation to a network model for the spread of sexually transmitted diseases. *Journal of Mathematical Biology*, 45(5):375–395.

Bauch, C. (2005). The spread of infectious diseases in spatially structured populations: An invasory pair approximation. *Mathematical Biosciences*, 198:217–237.

Bauch, C. and Rand, D. A. (2001). A moment closure model for sexually transmitted disease transmission through a concurrent partnership network. *Proceedings of the Royal Society of London, Series B, Biological Sciences*, 267(1485):2019–2027.

Bauch, C. T. and Earn, D. J. (2003). Transients and attractors in epidemics. *Proceedings of the Royal Society of London, Series B, Biological Sciences*, 270(1524):1573–1578.

Bauch, C. T., Lloyd-Smith, J. O., Coffee, M. P., and Galvani, A. P. (2005). Dynamically modeling SARS and other newly emerging respiratory illnesses — past, present, and future. *Epidemiology*, 16(6):791–801.

Becker, N. G. (1989). *Analysis of Infectious Disease Data*. Chapman and Hall, London.

Becker, N. G. (1993). Martingale methods for the analysis of epidemic data. *Statistical Methods in Medical Research*, 2(1):93–112.

Becker, N. G. and Hopper, J. L. (1983). Assessing the heterogeneity of disease spread through a community. *American Journal of Epidemiology*, 117(3):362–374.

Becker, N. G. and Marschner, I. (1990). The effect of heterogeneity on the spread of disease. In Gabriel, J.-P., Lefévre, C., and Picard, P., editors, *Stochastic Processes in Epidemic Theory*, Lecture Notes in Biomathematics 86, pages 90–103. Springer-Verlag, New York.

Begon, M., Bennett, M., Bowers, R. G., French, N. P., Hazel, S. M., and Turner, J. (2002). A clarification of transmission terms in host-microparasite models: Numbers, densities and areas. *Epidemiology and Infection*, 129:147–153.

Bell, D. M. and WGICTS (2004). Public health interventions and SARS spread, 2003. *Emerging Infectious Diseases*, 10(11):1900–1906. WGICTS = World Health Organization Working Group on International and Community Transmission of SARS.

Belova, L. A., Vasilyeva, V. I., Rvachev, L. A., and et al. (1982). New influenza epidemic model for the USSR territory (in Russian). Presented at the Seventh International Symposium on Influenza, Leningrad.

Bickerstaff, K. and Simmons, P. (2004). The right tool for the job? Modeling, spatial relationships, and styles of scientific practice in the UK foot and mouth crisis. *Environment and Planning D, Society and Space*, 22:393–412.

Bjørnstad, O. N., Finkenstädt, B. F., and Grenfell, B. T. (2002). Dynamics of measles epidemics: Estimating scaling of transmission rates using a time series SIR model. *Ecological Monographs*, 72(2):169–184.

Black, F. L. (1966). Measles endemicity in insular populations: Critical community size and its evolutionary implication. *Journal of Theoretical Biology*, 11:207–211.

Blythe, S. P. and Anderson, R. M. (1988). Variable infectiousness in HIV transmission models. *IMA Journal of Mathematics Applied in Medicine and Biology*, 5:181–200.

Blythe, S. P. and Castillo-Chavez, C. (1989). Like-with-like preference and sexual mixing models. *Mathematical Biosciences*, 96(2):221–238.

Blythe, S. P., Castillo-Chavez, C., Palmer, J., and Cheng, M. (1991). Towards unified theory of mixing and pair formation. *Mathematical Biosciences*, 107:379–405.

Bolker, B. M. and Grenfell, B. T. (1993). Chaos and biological complexity in measles dynamics. *Proceedings of the Royal Society of London, Series B, Biological Sciences*, 251(1330):75–81.

Bolker, B. M. and Grenfell, B. T. (1995). Space, persistence and dynamics of measles epidemics. *Philosophical Transactions of the Royal Society of London, Series B, Biological Sciences*, 348(1325):309–320.

Bolker, B. M. and Grenfell, B. T. (1996). Impact of vaccination on the spatial correlation and persistence of measles dynamics. *Proceedings of the National Academy of Sciences of the United States of America*, 93(22):12648–12653.

Bolker, B. M. and Pacala, S. W. (1997). Using moment equations to understand stochastically driven spatial pattern formation in ecological systems. *Theoretical Population Biology*, 52(3):179–197.

Bollobás, B. (1985). *Random Graphs*. Academic Press, London.

Bonabeau, E., Toubiana, L., and Flahault, A. (1998). The geographical spread of influenza. *Proceedings of the Royal Society of London, Series B, Biological Sciences*, 265(1413):2421–2425.

Boone, J. D., McGwire, K. C., Otteson, E. W., DeBaca, R. S., Kuhn, E. A., Villard, P., Brussard, P. F., and St Jeor, S. C. (2000). Remote sensing and geographic information systems: Charting Sin Nombre virus infections in deer mice. *Emerging Infectious Diseases*, 6(3):248–258.

Brauer, F. and Castillo-Chavez, C. (2001). *Mathematical Models in Population Biology and Epidemiology*. Springer-Verlag, New York.

Breugelmans, J. G., Zucs, P., Porten, K., Broll, S., Niedrig, M., Ammon, A., and Krause, G. (2004). SARS transmission and commercial aircraft. *Emerging Infectious Diseases*, 10(8):1502–1503.

Brimblecombe, F. S. W., Cruickshank, R., Masters, F. W., Reid, D. D., and Stewart, G. T. (1958). Family studies of respiratory infections. *British Medical Journal*, 1:119–128.

Broadbent, S. R. and Hammersley, J. M. (1957). Percolation processes, I: Crystals and mazes. *Proceedings of the Cambridge Philosophical Society*, 53:629–641.

Brockmann, D., Hufnagel, L., and Geisel, T. (2006). The scaling laws of human travel. *Nature*, 439:462–465.

Bron, C. and Kerbosch, J. (1973). Finding all cliques of an undirected graph — algorithm. *Communications of the ACM*, 16:575–577.

Brownstein, J. S., Wolfe, C. J., and Mandl, K. D. (2006). Empirical evidence for the effect of airline travel on inter-regional influenza spread in the United States. *PLOS Medicine*, 3(10):1826–1835.

Busenberg, S. N. and Castillo-Chavez, C. (1991). A general solution of the problem of mixing sub-populations, and its application to risk- and age-structured epidemic models for the spread of AIDS. *IMA Journal of Mathematics Applied in Medicine and Biology*, 8:1–29.

Cairns, A. J. (1990). Epidemics in heterogeneous populations, II: Non-exponential incubation periods and variable infectiousness. *IMA Journal of Mathematics Applied in Medicine and Biology*, 7(4):219–230.

Carrat, F. and Valleron, A. J. (1992). Epidemiologic mapping using the "kriging" method: Application to an influenza-like illness epidemic in France. *American Journal of Epidemiology*, 135(11):1293–1300.

Castillo-Chavez, C. and Busenberg, S. N. (1990). On the solution of the two-sex mixing problem. In Busenberg, S. N. and Martelli, M., editors, *Proceedings of the International Conference on Differential Equations and Applications to Biology and Population Dynamics*, Lecture Notes in Biomathematics 92, pages 80–98. Springer-Verlag, New York.

Castillo-Chavez, C., Cooke, K., Huang, W., and Levin, S. A. (1989a). On the role of long incubation periods in the dynamics of acquired immunodeficiency syndrome (AIDS), part 1: Single population models. *Journal of Mathematical Biology*, 27(4):373–398.

Castillo-Chavez, C., Cooke, K., Huang, W., and Levin, S. A. (1989b). The role of long incubation periods in the dynamics of HIV/AIDS, part 2: Multiple group models. In Castillo-Chavez, C., editor, *Mathematical and Statistical Approaches to AIDS Epidemiology*, Lecture Notes in Biomathematics 83, pages 200–217. Springer-Verlag, New York.

Cayley, A. L. (1857). On the theory of analytical forms called trees. *Philosophical Magazine*, 13:19–30. Reprinted in *Mathematical Papers, Cambridge*, 3:242-246, 1891.

Cayley, A. L. (1874). On the mathematical theory of isomers. *Philosophical Magazine*, 67:444–446. Reprinted in *Mathematical Papers, Cambridge*, 9:202-204, 1895.

Chaput, E. K., Meek, J. I., and Heimer, R. (2002). Spatial analysis of human granulocytic ehrlichiosis near Lyme, Connecticut. *Emerging Infectious Diseases*, 8(9):943–948.

Chau, P. H. and Yip, P. S. (2003). Monitoring the severe acute respiratory syndrome epidemic and assessing effectiveness of interventions in Hong Kong Special Administrative Region. *Journal of Epidemiology and Community Health*, 57(10):766–769.

Chick, S. E., Adams, A. L., and Koopman, J. S. (2000). Analysis and simulation of a stochastic, discrete-individual model of STD transmission with partnership concurrency. *Mathematical Biosciences*, 166(1):45–68.

Chowell, G., Castillo-Chavez, C., Fenimore, P. W., Kribs-Zaleta, C. M., Arriola, L., and Hyman, J. M. (2004). Model parameters and outbreak control for SARS. *Emerging Infectious Diseases*, 10(7):1258–1263.

Chowell, G., Fenimore, P. W., Castillo-Garsow, M. A., and Castillo-

Chavez, C. (2003). SARS outbreaks in Ontario, Hong Kong and Singapore: The role of diagnosis and isolation as a control mechanism. *Journal of Theoretical Biology*, 224:1–8.

Chung, F. and Lu, L. (2001). The diameter of random sparse graphs. *Advances in Applied Mathematics*, 26:257–279.

Chung, F. and Lu, L. (2002). The average distances in random graphs with given expected degrees. *Proceedings of the National Academy of Sciences of the United States of America*, 99(25):15879–15882.

Clarke, K. C., McLafferty, S. L., and Tempalski, B. J. (1996). On epidemiology and geographic information systems: A review and discussion of future directions. *Emerging Infectious Diseases*, 2(2):85–92.

Cliff, A. D. (1995). Analysing geographically-related disease data. *Statistical Methods in Medical Research*, 4(2):93–101.

Cliff, A. D. and Haggett, P. (1980). Changes in the seasonal incidence of measles in Iceland, 1896-1974. *Journal of Hygiene–Cambridge*, 85(3):451–457.

Cliff, A. D. and Haggett, P. (1983). Changing urban-rural contrasts in the velocity of measles epidemics in an island community. In McGlashan, N., editor, *Geographical Aspects of Health: Essays in Honour of Andrew Learmonth*, pages 335–348. Academic Press, London.

Cliff, A. D. and Haggett, P. (1984). Island epidemics. *Scientific American*, 250(5):138–147.

Cliff, A. D. and Haggett, P. (1985). *The Spread of Measles in Fiji and the Pacific: Spatial Components in the Transmission of Epidemic Waves Through Island Communities*. Australian National University, Canberra.

Cliff, A. D. and Haggett, P. (1988). *Atlas of Disease Distributions*. Blackwell, Oxford.

Cliff, A. D. and Haggett, P. (1993). Statistical modelling of measles and influenza outbreaks. *Statistical Methods in Medical Research*, 2(1):43–73.

Cliff, A. D., Haggett, P., and Graham, R. (1983a). Reconstruction of diffusion processes at local scales: The 1846, 1882 and 1904 measles epidemics in northwest Iceland. *Journal of Historical Geography*, 9(4):347–368.

Cliff, A. D., Haggett, P., and Ord, J. K. (1983b). Forecasting epidemic pathways for measles in Iceland: The use of simultaneous equation and logit models. *Ecology of Disease*, 2(4):377–396.

Cliff, A. D., Haggett, P., Ord, J. K., and Versey, J. R. (1981). *Spa-*

tial Diffusion: An Historical Geography of Epidemics in an Island Community. Cambridge University Press, Cambridge.

Cliff, A. D., Haggett, P., and Smallman-Raynor, M. R. (1993). *Measles: An Historical Geography of a Major Human Viral Disease from Global Expansion to Local Retreat, 1840-1990*. Blackwell, London.

Cliff, A. D., Haggett, P., Smallman-Raynor, M. R., Stroup, D. F., and Williamson, G. D. (1995). The application of multidimensional scaling methods to epidemiological data. *Statistical Methods in Medical Research*, 4(2):102–123.

Cliff, A. D., Haggett, P., and Stroup, D. F. (1992a). The geographic structure of measles epidemics in the northeastern United States. *American Journal of Epidemiology*, 136(5):592–602.

Cliff, A. D., Haggett, P., Stroup, D. F., and Cheney, E. (1992b). The changing geographical coherence of measles morbidity in the United States, 1962-88. *Statistics in Medicine*, 11(11):1409–1424.

Cliff, A. D. and Ord, J. K. (1978). Forecasting the progress of an epidemic. In Martin, R. L., Thrift, N. J., and Bennett, R. J., editors, *Towards the Dynamic Analysis of Spatial Systems*, pages 191–204. Pion, London.

Cliff, A. D. and Ord, J. K. (1985). Forecasting the spread of an epidemic. In Anderson, O. D., Ord, J. K., and Robinson, E. A., editors, *Time Series Analysis, Theory and Practice 6: Hydrological, Geophysical, and Spatial Applications*, pages 297–308. North-Holland, Amsterdam.

Cockburn, T. A. (1971). Infectious diseases in ancient populations. *Current Anthropology*, 12:45–62.

Colizza, V., Barrat, A., Barthelemy, M., and Vespignani, A. (2006a). The modeling of global epidemics: Stochastic dynamics and predictability. *Bulletin of Mathematical Biology*, 68(8):1893–1921.

Colizza, V., Barrat, A., Barthelemy, M., and Vespignani, A. (2006b). The role of the airline transportation network in the prediction and predictability of global epidemics. *Proceedings of the National Academy of Sciences of the United States of America*, 103(7):2051–2020.

Cooke, K. L., Calef, D. F., and Level, E. V. (1977). Stability or chaos in discrete epidemic models. In Lakshmikantham, V., editor, *Nonlinear Systems and Applications*, pages 73–93. Academic Press, New York.

Cooper, B. S., Pitman, R. J., Edmunds, W. J., and Gay, N. J. (2006).

Delaying the international spread of pandemic influenza. *PLOS Medicine*, 3(6):845–855.

Cox, D. R. and Miller, H. D. (1965). *The Theory of Stochastic Processes*. Wiley, New York.

Cox, S. J., Barnett, P. V., Dani, P., and Salt, J. S. (1999). Emergency vaccination of sheep against foot-and-mouth disease: Protection against disease and reduction in contact transmission. *Vaccine*, 17(15-16):1858–1868.

Crosby, A. W. (1989). *America's Forgotten Pandemic: The Influenza of 1918*. Cambridge University Press, New York.

Cushing, J. M. (1998). *An Introduction to Structured Population Dynamics*. CBMS-NSF Regional Conference Series in Applied Mathematics 71. Society for Industrial and Applied Mathematics, Philadelphia.

Daniels, H. E. (1977). The advancing wave in a spatial birth process. *Journal of Applied Probability*, 14:689–701.

Davies, G. (2002). Foot and mouth disease. *Research in Veterinary Science*, 73(3):195–199.

Davis, A., Gardner, B. B., and Gardner, M. R. (1941). *Deep South*. University of Chicago Press, Chicago.

Davis, J. A. and Leinhardt, S. (1972). The structure of positive interpersonal relations in small groups. In Berger, J., Zelditch, Jr., M., and Anderson, B., editors, *Sociological Theories in Progress, Volume II*, pages 218–251. Houghton Mifflin, Boston.

de Jong, M. C. M., Diekmann, O., and Heesterbeek, J. A. P. (1995). How does transmission of infection depend on population size? In Mollison, D., editor, *Epidemic Models: Their Structure and Relation to Data*, pages 84–94. Cambridge University Press, Cambridge.

DeAngelis, D. L. and Gross, L. J. (1992). *Individual-based Models and Approaches in Ecology: Populations, Communities, and Ecosystems*. Chapman and Hall, New York.

Diekmann, O. (1978). Thresholds and travelling waves for the geographical spread of infection. *Journal of Mathematical Biology*, 6(2):109–130.

Diekmann, O., de Jong, M. C. M., and Metz, J. A. J. (1998a). A deterministic epidemic model taking account of repeated contacts between the same individuals. *Journal of Applied Probability*, 35:448–462.

Diekmann, O., Gyllenberg, M., Metz, J. A., and Thieme, H. R. (1998b). On the formulation and analysis of general deterministic structured population models, I: Linear theory. *Journal of Mathematical Biology*, 36:349–388.

Diekmann, O. and Heesterbeek, J. A. P. (2000). *Mathematical Epidemiology of Infectious Diseases: Model Building, Analysis, and Interpretation*. John Wiley, New York.

Diekmann, O., Heesterbeek, J. A. P., and Metz, J. A. J. (1990). On the definition and the computation of the basic reproduction rate R_0 in models for infectious diseases in heterogeneous populations. *Journal of Mathematical Biology*, 28:365–382.

Diekmann, O., Heesterbeek, J. A. P., and Metz, J. A. J. (1995). The legacy of Kermack and McKendrick. In Mollison, D., editor, *Epidemic Models: Their Structure and Relation to Data*, Publications of the Newton Institute, pages 95–115. Cambridge University Press, Cambridge.

Dietz, K. (1980). Models for vector-borne parasitic diseases. In Berigozzi, C., editor, *Vito Volterra Symposium on Mathematical Models in Biology*, Lecture Notes in Biomathematics 39, pages 264–277. Springer-Verlag, Berlin.

Dietz, K. (1982). Overall patterns in the transmission cycle of infectious disease agents. In Anderson, R. M. and May, R. M., editors, *Population Biology of Infectious Diseases*, pages 87–102. Springer-Verlag, Berlin.

Dietz, K. (1988). The first epidemic model: A historical note on P. D. En'ko. *Australian Journal of Statistics*, 30A:56–65.

Dietz, K. and Hadeler, K. P. (1988). Epidemiological models for sexually transmitted diseases. *Journal of Mathematical Biology*, 26:1–25.

Dietz, K. and Schenzle, D. (1985). Mathematical models for infectious disease statistics. In Atkinson, A. C. and Feinberg, S. E., editors, *A Celebration of Statistics: The ISI Centenary Volume*, pages 167–204. Springer-Verlag, New York.

Doel, T. R., Williams, L., and Barnett, P. V. (1994). Emergency vaccination against foot-and-mouth disease: Rate of development of immunity and its implications for the carrier state. *Vaccine*, 12(7):592–600.

Doering, C. R. (1991). Modeling complex systems: Stochastic processes, stochastic differential equations, and Fokker-Planck equations. In Nadel, L. and Stein, D. L., editors, *1990 Lectures in Complex Systems: The Proceedings of the 1990 Complex Systems Summer School, Santa Fe, New Mexico, June 1990*, Santa Fe Institute Studies in the Sciences of Complexity, Lectures v. 3. Addison-

Wesley, Redwood City, CA.

Doherty, I. A., Shiboski, S., Ellen, J. M., Adimora, A. A., and Padian, N. S. (2006). Sexual bridging socially and over time: A simulation model exploring the relative effects of mixing and concurrency on viral sexually transmitted infection transmission. *Sexually Transmitted Diseases*, 33:368–373.

Donnelly, C. A., Ghani, A. C., Leung, G. M., Hedley, A. J., Fraser, C., Riley, S., Abu-Raddad, L. J., Ho, L. M., Thach, T. Q., Chau, P., Chan, K. P., Lam, T. H., Tse, L. Y., Tsang, T., Liu, S. H., Kong, J. H., Lau, E. M., Ferguson, N. M., and Anderson, R. M. (2003). Epidemiological determinants of spread of causal agent of severe acute respiratory syndrome in Hong Kong. *Lancet*, 361(9371):1761–1766.

Dorolle, P. (1968). Old plagues in the jet age: International aspects of present and future control of communicable disease. *British Medical Journal*, 4:789–792.

Dunn, F. L., Carey, D. E., Cohen, A., and Martin, J. D. (1959). Epidemiologic studies of Asian influenza in a Louisiana parish. *American Journal of Hygiene*, 70:351–371.

Dushoff, J., Plotkin, J. B., Viboud, C., Simonsen, L., Miller, M., Loeb, M., and Earn, D. J. D. (2007). Vaccinating to protect a vulnerable subpopulation. *PLOS Medicine*, 4(5):0921–0927.

Dye, C. and Gay, N. (2003). Modeling the SARS epidemic. *Science*, 300:1884–1885.

Dye, C. and Hasibeder, G. (1986). Population dynamics of mosquito-borne disease: Effects of flies which bite some people more frequently than others. *Transactions of the Royal Society of Tropical Medicine and Hygiene*, 80:69–77.

Eames, K. T. and Keeling, M. J. (2002). Modeling dynamic and network heterogeneities in the spread of sexually transmitted diseases. *Proceedings of the National Academy of Sciences of the United States of America*, 99(20):13330–13335.

Earn, D. J. D. and Levin, S. A. (2006). Global asymptotic coherence in discrete dynamical systems. *Proceedings of the National Academy of Sciences of the United States of America*, 103(11):3968–3971.

Earn, D. J. D., Levin, S. A., and Rohani, P. (2000a). Coherence and conservation. *Science*, 290(5495):1360–1364.

Earn, D. J. D., Rohani, P., Bolker, B. M., and Grenfell, B. T. (2000b). A simple model for complex dynamical transitions in epidemics. *Science*, 287(5453):667–670.

Eguiluz, V. M. and Klemm, K. (2002). Epidemic threshold in structured scale-free networks. *Physical Review Letters*, 89(10):108701.

Ellner, S. P. (2001). Pair approximation for lattice models with multiple interaction scales. *Journal of Theoretical Biology*, 210(4):435–447.

Ellner, S. P., Bailey, B. A., Bobashev, G. V., Gallant, A. R., Grenfell, B. T., and Nychka, D. W. (1998a). Noise and nonlinearity in measles epidemics: Combining mechanistic and statistical approaches to population modeling. *American Naturalist*, 151(5):425–440.

Ellner, S. P., Sasaki, A., Haraguchi, Y., and Matsuda, H. (1998b). Speed of invasion in lattice population models: Pair-edge approximation. *Journal of Mathematical Biology*, 36:469–484.

Elveback, L., Ackerman, E., Gatewood, L. G., and Fox, J. P. (1971). Stochastic two-agent epidemic simulation models for a community of families. *American Journal of Epidemiology*, 93(4):267–280.

Elveback, L. R., Fox, J. P., Ackerman, E., Langworthy, A., Boyd, M., and Gatewood, L. G. (1976). An influenza simulation model for immunization studies. *American Journal of Epidemiology*, 103:152–165.

En'ko, P. D. (1889). On the course of epidemics of some infectious diseases. *Vrach St. Petersburg*, 10:1008–1010, 1039–1042, 1061–1063.

Eubank, S., Guclu, H., Kumar, A., Marathe, M. V., Srinivasan, A., Toroczkai, Z., and Wang, N. (2004). Modelling disease outbreaks in realistic urban social networks. *Nature*, 429(6988):180–184.

Ewy, W., Ackerman, E., Gatewood, L. G., Elveback, L., and Fox, J. P. (1972). A generalized stochastic model for simulation of epidemics in a heterogeneous population (Model VI). *Computers in Biology and Medicine*, 2:45–58.

Fararo, T. J. and Sunshine, M. (1989). *A Study of a Biased Friendship Network*. Syracuse University Press, Syracuse, NY.

Feld, S. L. (1991). Why your friends have more friends than you do. *American Journal of Sociology*, 96:1464–1477.

Ferguson, N. M., Cummings, D. A. T., Cauchemez, S., Fraser, C., Riley, S., Meeyai, A., Iamsirithaworn, S., and Burke, D. S. (2005). Strategies for containing an emerging influenza pandemic in Southeast Asia. *Nature*, 437(7056):209–214.

Ferguson, N. M., Cummings, D. A. T., Fraser, C., Cajka, J. C., Cooley, P. C., and Burke, D. S. (2006). Strategies for mitigating an influenza pandemic. *Nature*, 442:448–451.

Ferguson, N. M., Donnelly, C. A., and Anderson, R. M. (2001a). The foot-and-mouth epidemic in Great Britain: Pattern of spread and impact of interventions. *Science*, 292(5519):1155–1160.

Ferguson, N. M., Donnelly, C. A., and Anderson, R. M. (2001b). Transmission intensity and impact of control policies on the foot and mouth epidemic in Great Britain. *Nature*, 413(6855):542–548.

Ferguson, N. M., May, R. M., and Anderson, R. M. (1997). Measles: Persistence and synchronicity in disease dynamics and interspecific interactions. In Tilman, D. and Kareiva, P. M., editors, *Spatial Ecology: The Role of Space in Population Dynamics and Interspecific Interactions*, pages 137–157. Princeton University Press, Princeton, NJ.

Ferguson, N. M., Nokes, D. J., and Anderson, R. M. (1996). Dynamical complexity in age-structured models of the transmission of the measles virus: Epidemiological implications at high levels of vaccine uptake. *Mathematical Biosciences*, 138(2):101–130.

Ferrari, M. J., Grais, R. F., Bharti, N., Conlan, A. J. K., Bjørnstad, O. N., Wolfson, L. J., Guerin, P. J., Djibo, A., and Grenfell, B. T. (2008). The dynamics of measles in sub-Saharan Africa. *Nature*, 451:679–684.

Fiennes, R. (1978). *Zoonoses and the Origins and Ecology of Human Disease*. Academic Press, London.

Fine, P. E. (1982). Applications of mathematical models to the epidemiology of influenza: A critique. In Selby, P., editor, *Influenza Models: Prospects for Development and Use*, pages 15–85. MTP Press Limited, Lancaster.

Fine, P. E. and Clarkson, J. A. (1982). Measles in England and Wales, I: An analysis of factors underlying seasonal patterns. *International Journal of Epidemiology*, 11(1):5–14.

Fine, P. E. M. (2003). The interval between successive cases of an infectious disease. *American Journal of Epidemiology*, 158(11):1039–1047.

Finkenstädt, B. F. and Grenfell, B. T. (1998). Empirical determinants of measles metapopulation dynamics in England and Wales. *Proceedings of the Royal Society of London, Series B, Biological Sciences*, 265(1392):211–220.

Finkenstädt, B. F. and Grenfell, B. T. (2000). Time series modelling of childhood diseases: A dynamical systems approach. *Journal of the Royal Statistical Society, Series C, Applied Statistics*, 49:187–205.

Fisher, R. A. (1937). The wave of advance of advantageous genes.

Annals of Eugenics, 7:355–369.

Flahault, A., Deguen, S., and Valleron, A. J. (1994). A mathematical model for the European spread of influenza. *European Journal of Epidemiology*, 10(4):471–474.

Flahault, A., Letrait, S., Blin, P., Hazout, S., Menares, J., and Valleron, A. J. (1988). Modelling the 1985 influenza epidemic in France. *Statistics in Medicine*, 7(11):1147–1155.

Flahault, A., Vergu, E., Coudeville, L., and Grais, R. F. (2006). Strategies for containing a global influenza pandemic. *Vaccine*, 24(44-46):6751–6755.

Freeman, R. (2002). *A mathematical model for the geographic spread of infectious disease via air travel*. PhD thesis, Johns Hopkins University.

Fulford, G. R., Roberts, M. G., and Heesterbeek, J. A. P. (2002). The metapopulation dynamics of an infectious disease: Tuberculosis in possums. *Theoretical Population Biology*, 61(1):15–29.

Gani, R. and Leach, S. (2001). Transmission potential of smallpox in contemporary populations. *Nature*, 414(6865):748–751.

Gardner, L. I., Brundage, J. F., Burke, D. S., McNeil, J. G., Visintine, R., and Miller, R. N. (1989). Spatial diffusion of the human immunodeficiency virus infection epidemic in the United States, 1985-1987. *Annals of the Association of American Geographers*, 79:25–43.

Gatrell, A. C., Bailey, T. C., Diggle, P. J., and Rowlingson, B. S. (1996). Spatial point pattern analysis and its application in geographical epidemiology. *Transactions of the Institute of British Geographers*, 21(1):256–274.

Gatrell, A. C. and Löytönen, M. (1998). GIS and health research: An introduction. In Gatrell, A. C. and Löytönen, M., editors, *GIS and Health*, pages 3–16. Taylor and Francis, Philadelphia.

Germann, T. C., Kadau, K., Longini, Jr., I. M., and Macken, C. A. (2006). Mitigation strategies for pandemic influenza in the United States. *Proceedings of the National Academy of Sciences of the United States of America*, 103(15):5935–5940.

Ghani, A. C., Donnelly, C. A., and Garnett, G. P. (1998). Sampling biases and missing data in explorations of sexual partner networks for the spread of sexually transmitted diseases. *Statistics in Medicine*, 17:2079–2097.

Ghani, A. C. and Garnett, G. P. (1998). Measuring sexual partner networks for transmission of sexually transmitted diseases. *Journal of the Royal Statistical Society, Series A, Statistics in Society*,

161:227–238.

Ghani, A. C. and Garnett, G. P. (2000). Risks of acquiring and transmitting sexually transmitted diseases in sexual partner networks. *Sexually Transmitted Diseases*, 27(10):579–587.

Gibbens, J. C., Sharpe, C. E., Wilesmith, J. W., Mansley, L. M., Michalopoulou, E., Ryan, J. B., and Hudson, M. (2001). Descriptive epidemiology of the 2001 foot-and-mouth disease epidemic in Great Britain: The first five months. *Veterinary Record*, 149(24):729–743.

Gibson, M. A. and Bruck, J. (2000). Efficient exact stochastic simulation of chemical systems with many species and many channels. *Journal of Physical Chemistry A*, 104:1876–1889.

Gillespie, D. T. (1977). Exact stochastic simulation of coupled chemical reactions. *Journal of Physical Chemistry A*, 81:2340–2361.

Girvan, M., Callaway, D. S., Newman, M. E. J., and Strogatz, S. H. (2002). A simple model of epidemics with pathogen mutation. *Physical Review E*, 63:031915.

Glavanakov, S., White, D. J., Caraco, T., Lapenis, A., Robinson, G. R., Szymanski, B. K., and Maniatty, W. A. (2001). Lyme disease in New York State: Spatial pattern at a regional scale. *American Journal of Tropical Medicine and Hygiene*, 65(5):538–545.

Glezen, W. P. (1996). Emerging infections: Pandemic influenza. *Epidemiologic Reviews*, 18:64–76.

Gloster, J., Blackall, R. M., Sellers, R. F., and Donaldson, A. I. (1981). Forecasting the airborne spread of foot-and-mouth disease. *Veterinary Record*, 108(17):370–374.

Golub, A., Gorr, W. L., and Gould, P. R. (1993). Spatial diffusion of the HIV/AIDS epidemic: Modeling implications and case study of AIDS incidence in Ohio. *Geographical Analysis*, 25(2):85–100.

Gould, P. R. (1989). Geographic dimension of the AIDS epidemic. *Professional Geographer*, 41:71–78.

Gould, P. R., Kabel, J., Gorr, W. L., and Golub, A. (1991). AIDS: Predicting the next map. *Interfaces*, 21(3):80–92.

Grais, R. F., Ellis, J. H., and Glass, G. E. (2003). Assessing the impact of airline travel on the geographic spread of pandemic influenza. *European Journal of Epidemiology*, 18(11):1065–1072.

Grais, R. F., Ellis, J. H., Kress, A., and Glass, G. E. (2004). Modeling the spread of annual influenza epidemics in the U.S.: The potential role of air travel. *Health Care Management Science*, 7(2):127–134.

Granovetter, M. S. (1973). The strength of weak ties. *American*

Journal of Sociology, 78:1360–1380.

Grassberger, P. (1983). On the critical behavior of the general epidemic process and dynamical percolation. *Mathematical Biosciences*, 63:157–172.

Gray, R. H., Wawer, M. J., Brookmeyer, R., Sewankambo, N. K., Serwadda, D., Wabwire-Mangen, F., Lutalo, T., Lin, X., vanCott, T., Quinn, T. C., and the Rakai Project Team (2001). Probability of HIV-1 transmission per coital act in monogamous, heterosexual, HIV-1-discordant couples in Rakai, Uganda. *Lancet*, 357:1149–1153.

Green, L. E. and Medley, G. F. (2002). Mathematical modelling of the foot and mouth disease epidemic of 2001: Strengths and weaknesses. *Research in Veterinary Science*, 73(3):201–205.

Greenwood, M. (1931). On the statistical measure of infectiousness. *Journal of Hygiene–Cambridge*, 31:336–351.

Grenfell, B. T. (1992). Chance and chaos in measles dynamics. *Journal of the Royal Statistical Society, Series B, Statistical Methodology*, 54(2):383–398.

Grenfell, B. T. (2002). Rivers dam waves of rabies. *Proceedings of the National Academy of Sciences of the United States of America*, 99(6):3365–3367.

Grenfell, B. T., Bjørnstad, O. N., and Finkenstädt, B. F. (2002). Dynamics of measles epidemics: Scaling noise, determinism, and predictability with the TSIR model. *Ecological Monographs*, 72(2):185–202.

Grenfell, B. T., Bjørnstad, O. N., and Kappey, J. (2001). Travelling waves and spatial hierarchies in measles epidemics. *Nature*, 414(6865):716–723.

Grenfell, B. T. and Bolker, B. M. (1998). Cities and villages: Infection hierarchies in a measles metapopulation. *Ecology Letters*, 1(1):63–70.

Grenfell, B. T. and Harwood, J. (1997). (Meta)population dynamics of infectious diseases. *Trends in Ecology and Evolution*, 12(10):395–399.

Grimmett, G. (1999). *Percolation*. Grundlehren der Mathematischen Wissenschaften 321. Springer, New York, 2nd edition.

Grossman, Z. (1980). Oscillatory phenomena in a model of infectious diseases. *Theoretical Population Biology*, 18:204–243.

Guimerà, R. and Amaral, L. A. N. (2004). Modeling the world-wide airport network. *European Physical Journal B*, 38(2):381–385.

Gumel, A. B., Ruan, S., Day, T., Watmough, J., Brauer, F., van den Driessche, P., Gabrielson, D., Bowman, C., Alexander, M. E., Ardal, S., Wu, J., and Sahai, B. M. (2004). Modelling strategies for controlling SARS outbreaks. *Proceedings of the Royal Society of London, Series B, Biological Sciences*, 271(1554):2223–2232.

Gupta, S., Anderson, R. M., and May, R. M. (1989). Networks of sexual contacts: Implications for the pattern of spread of HIV. *AIDS*, 3:807–817.

Gwaltney Jr., J. M., Hendley, J. O., Simon, G., and Jordan Jr., W. S. (1966). Rhinovirus infections in an industrial population, I: The occurrence of illness. *New England Journal of Medicine*, 275(23):1261–1268.

Haggett, P. (1982). Building geographic components into epidemiological models. In Selby, P., editor, *Influenza Models*, pages 203–212. MTP Press Limited, Lancaster.

Haining, R. P. (2003). *Spatial Data Analysis: Theory and Practice*. Cambridge University Press, Cambridge.

Hamer, W. H. (1906). Epidemic disease in England — the evidence of variability and of persistency of type. *Lancet*, 1:733–739.

Hammersley, J. M. (1957). Percolation processes: Lower bounds for the critical probability. *Annals of Mathematics and Statistics*, 28:790–795.

Hammersley, J. M. (1959). Bornes superieures de la probabilite critique dans un process de filtration. In *Le Calcul des Probabilities et Ses Applications*, Paris, 15-20 Juillet, 1958. Centre National de la Recherche Scientifique (CNRS).

Hannay, D. and Jones, R. (2002). The effects of foot-and-mouth on the health of those involved in farming and tourism in Dumfries and Galloway. *European Journal of General Practice*, 8:83–89.

Harary, F. and Norman, R. Z. (1953). *Graph Theory as a Mathematical Model in Social Science*. University of Michigan Institute of Social Research, Ann Arbor.

Harary, F., Norman, R. Z., and Cartwright, D. (1965). *Structural Models: An Introduction to the Theory of Directed Graphs*. John Wiley & Sons, New York.

Harris, T. E. (1974). Contact interactions on a lattice. *Annals of Probability*, 2:969–988.

Hawryluk, L., Gold, W. L., Robinson, S., Pogorski, S., Galea, S., and Styra, R. (2004). SARS control and psychological effects of quarantine, Toronto, Canada. *Emerging Infectious Diseases*, 10(7):1206–

1212.

Haydon, D. T., Kao, R. R., and Kitching, R. P. (2004). The UK foot-and-mouth-disease outbreak — the aftermath. *Nature Reviews Microbiology*, 2(8):675–681.

He, D. H. and Stone, L. (2003). Spatio-temporal synchronization of recurrent epidemics. *Proceedings of the Royal Society of London, Series B, Biological Sciences*, 270(1523):1519–1526.

Heasman, M. A. and Reid, D. D. (1961). Theory and observation in family epidemics of the common cold. *British Journal of Preventive and Social Medicine*, 15:12–16.

Heesterbeek, J. A. P. and Dietz, K. (1996). The concept of R_0 in epidemic theory. *Statistica Neerlandica*, 50:89–110.

Heil, G. H. and White, H. C. (1976). An algorithm for finding simultaneous homomorphic correspondences between graphs and their image graphs. *Behavioral Science*, 21:26–35.

Hendley, J. O., Gwaltney Jr., J. M., and Jordan Jr., W. S. (1969). Rhinovirus infections in an industrial population, IV: Infections within families of employees during two fall peaks of respiratory illness. *American Journal of Epidemiology*, 89(2):184–196.

Herring, D. A. and Sattenspiel, L. (2003). Death in winter: The Spanish flu in the Canadian Subarctic. In Phillips, H. and Killingray, D., editors, *The Spanish Influenza Pandemic of 1918-19*, pages 156–172. Routledge, London.

Hethcote, H. W. (1974). Asymptotic behaviour and stability in epidemic models. In van den Driessche, P., editor, *Mathematical Problems in Biology*, Lecture Notes in Biomathematics 2, pages 83–92. Springer-Verlag, New York.

Hethcote, H. W. (1978). An immunization model for a heterogeneous population. *Theoretical Population Biology*, 14:338–349.

Hethcote, H. W. (1989). A model for HIV transmission and AIDS. In Castillo-Chavez, C., Levin, S. A., and Shoemaker, C., editors, *Mathematical Approaches to Resource Management and Epidemiology*, Lecture Notes in Biomathematics 81, pages 164–176. Springer-Verlag, Berlin.

Hethcote, H. W. (1998). Oscillations in an endemic model for pertussis. *Canadian Applied Mathematics Quarterly*, 6:61–88.

Hethcote, H. W. and Thieme, H. R. (1985). Stability of the endemic equilibrium in epidemic models with subpopulations. *Mathematical Biosciences*, 75:205–227.

Hethcote, H. W. and Tudor, D. W. (1980). Integral equation models for endemic infectious diseases. *Journal of Mathematical Biology*, 9(1):37–47.

Hethcote, H. W. and Van Ark, J. W. (1987). Epidemiological models for heterogeneous populations: Proportionate mixing, parameter estimation, and immunization programs. *Mathematical Biosciences*, 84:85–118.

Hethcote, H. W., Yorke, J. A., and Nold, A. (1982). Gonorrhea modelling: A comparison of control methods. *Mathematical Biosciences*, 58:93–109.

Heymann, D. L., editor (2004). *Control of Communicable Diseases Manual*. The American Public Health Association, Washington, DC, 18th edition.

Higham, D. J. (2001). An algorithmic introduction to numerical simulation of stochastic differential equations. *SIAM Review*, 43(3):525–546.

Hill, A. V., Allsopp, C. E., Kwiatkowski, D., Anstey, N. M., Twumasi, P., Rowe, P. A., Bennett, S., Brewster, D., McMichael, A. J., and Greenwood, B. M. (1991). Common West African HLA antigens are associated with protection from severe malaria. *Nature*, 352(6336):595–600.

Hilleman, M. R. (2002). Realities and enigmas of human viral influenza: Pathogenesis, epidemiology and control. *Vaccine*, 20:3068–3087.

Holland, P. W. and Leinhardt, S. (1971). Transitivity in structural models of small groups. *Comparative Group Studies*, 2:107–124.

Holland, P. W. and Leinhardt, S. (1976). Local structure in social networks. *Sociological Methodology*, 7:1–45.

Honhold, N., Taylor, N. M., Mansley, L. M., and Paterson, A. D. (2004). Relationship of speed of slaughter on infected premises and intensity of culling of other premises to the rate of spread of the foot-and-mouth disease epidemic in Great Britain, 2001. *Veterinary Record*, 155(10):287–294.

Hope Simpson, R. E. (1952). Infectiousness of communicable diseases in the household. *The Lancet*, 2:549–554.

Hoppensteadt, F. (1974). An age dependent epidemic model. *Journal of the Franklin Institute, Engineering and Applied Mathematics*, 297:325–333.

Hsieh, Y. H., Chen, C. W. S., and Hsu, S. B. (2004). SARS outbreak, Taiwan, 2003. *Emerging Infectious Diseases*, 10(2):201–206.

Hsieh, Y. H., King, C. C., Chen, C. W. S., Ho, M. S., Lee, J. Y.,

Liu, F. C., Wu, Y. C., and JulianWu, J. S. (2005). Quarantine for SARS, Taiwan. *Emerging Infectious Diseases*, 11(2):278–282.

Hufnagel, L., Brockmann, D., and Geisel, T. (2004). Forecast and control of epidemics in a globalized world. *Proceedings of the National Academy of Sciences of the United States of America*, 101(42):15124–15129.

Hugh-Jones, M. E. and Wright, P. B. (1970). Studies on the 1967-8 foot-and-mouth disease epidemic: The relation of weather to the spread of disease. *Journal of Hygiene–Cambridge*, 68(2):253–271.

Hyman, J. M. and LaForce, T. (2003). Modeling the spread of influenza among cities. In Banks, H. T. and Castillo-Chavez, C., editors, *Bioterrorism: Mathematical Modeling Applications in Homeland Security*, pages 211–236. Society for Industrial and Applied Mathematics, Philadelphia.

Hyman, J. M. and Stanley, E. A. (1988). Using mathematical models to understand the AIDS epidemic. *Mathematical Biosciences*, 90:415–474.

Isham, V. (1991). Assessing the variability of stochastic epidemics. *Mathematical Biosciences*, 107(2):209–224.

Jacquez, G. M., Grimson, R., Waller, L. A., and Wartenberg, D. (1996a). The analysis of disease clusters, part II: Introduction to techniques. *Infection Control and Hospital Epidemiology*, 17(6):385–397.

Jacquez, G. M., Waller, L. A., Grimson, R., and Wartenberg, D. (1996b). The analysis of disease clusters, part I: State of the art. *Infection Control and Hospital Epidemiology*, 17(5):319–327.

Jacquez, J. A. (1996). *Compartmental Models in Medicine and Biology*. BioMedware, Ann Arbor, MI, 3rd edition.

Jacquez, J. A., Koopman, J. S., Simon, C. P., Sattenspiel, L., and Perry, T. (1988). Modeling and analyzing HIV transmission: The effect of contact patterns. *Mathematical Biosciences*, 92:119–199.

Jagers, P. (1975). *Branching Processes with Biological Applications*. Wiley, New York.

Jalvingh, A. W., Nielen, M., Maurice, H., Stegeman, A. J., Elbers, A. R., and Dijkhuizen, A. A. (1999). Spatial and stochastic simulation to evaluate the impact of events and control measures on the 1997-1998 classical swine fever epidemic in the Netherlands, I: Description of simulation model. *Preventive Veterinary Medicine*, 42(3-4):271–295.

Jansen, V. A. A. and Lloyd, A. L. (2000). Local stability analysis of spatially homogeneous solutions of multi-patch systems. *Journal of Mathematical Biology*, 41(3):232–252.

Jeffery, K. J., Usuku, K., Hall, S. E., Matsumoto, W., Taylor, G. P., Procter, J., Bunce, M., Ogg, G. S., Welsh, K. I., Weber, J. N., Lloyd, A. L., Nowak, M. A., Nagai, M., Kodama, D., Izumo, S., Osame, M., and Bangham, C. R. (1999). HLA alleles determine human T-lymphotropic virus-I (HTLV-I) proviral load and the risk of HTLV-I-associated myelopathy. *Proceedings of the National Academy of Sciences of the United States of America*, 96(7):3848–3853.

Jeltsch, F., Muller, M. S., Grimm, V., Wissel, C., and Brandl, R. (1997). Pattern formation triggered by rare events: Lessons from the spread of rabies. *Proceedings of the Royal Society of London, Series B, Biological Sciences*, 264(1381):495–503.

Jensen, A. (1948). An elucidation of Erlang's statistical works through the theory of stochastic processes. In Brockmeyer, E., Halstrøm, H. L., and Jensen, A., editors, *The Life and Works of A. K. Erlang*, pages 23–100. The Copenhagen Telephone Company, Copenhagen.

Johnson, N. P. A. S. and Mueller, J. (2002). Updating the accounts: Global mortality of the 1918-1920 "Spanish" influenza pandemic. *Bulletin of the History of Medicine*, 76:105–115.

Jones, J. H. and Handcock, M. S. (2003). Sexual contacts and epidemic thresholds. *Nature*, 423:605–606.

Jorde, L. B., Pitkänen, K., Mielke, J. H., Fellman, J. O., and Eriksson, A. W. (1990). Historical epidemiology of smallpox in Kitee, Finland. In Swedlund, A. C. and Armelagos, G., editors, *The Health and Disease of Populations in Transition*, pages 183–200. Bergin & Garvey, New York.

Kao, R. R. (2002). The role of mathematical modelling in the control of the 2001 FMD epidemic in the UK. *Trends in Microbiology*, 10(6):279–286.

Kao, R. R. (2003). The impact of local heterogeneity on alternative control strategies for foot-and-mouth disease. *Proceedings of the Royal Society of London, Series B, Biological Sciences*, 270(1533):2557–2564.

Kaplan, E. H. (1989). Can bad models suggest good policies? Sexual mixing and the AIDS epidemic. *Journal of Sex Research*, 26:301–314.

Kaplan, E. H. and Lee, Y. S. (1990). How bad can it get? Bounding worst case endemic heterogeneous mixing models of HIV/AIDS.

Mathematical Biosciences, 99:157–180.

Kaplan, M. and Webster, R. G. (1977). The epidemiology of influenza. *Scientific American*, 237(6):88–106.

Karatzas, I. and Shreve, S. E. (1991). *Brownian Motion and Stochastic Calculus*. Graduate Texts in Mathematics 113. Springer-Verlag, New York, 2nd edition.

Karinthy, F. (1929). Chains. In *Everything is the Other Way*. Atheneum Press, Budapest.

Keeling, M., Tildesley, M., Savill, N., Woolhouse, M., Shaw, D., Deardon, R., Brooks, S., and Grenfell, B. (2006). FMD control strategies (reply). *Veterinary Record*, 158(20):707–708.

Keeling, M. J. (1999a). Correlation equations for endemic diseases: Externally imposed and internally generated heterogeneity. *Proceedings of the Royal Society of London, Series B, Biological Sciences*, 266(1422):953–960.

Keeling, M. J. (1999b). The effects of local spatial structure on epidemiological invasions. *Proceedings of the Royal Society of London, Series B, Biological Sciences*, 266(1421):859–867.

Keeling, M. J. (2000a). Metapopulation moments: Coupling, stochasticity and persistence. *Journal of Animal Ecology*, 69(5):725–736.

Keeling, M. J. (2000b). Multiplicative moments and measures of persistence in ecology. *Journal of Theoretical Biology*, 205(2):269–281.

Keeling, M. J. (2005). Models of foot-and-mouth disease. *Proceedings of the Royal Society of London, Series B, Biological Sciences*, 272(1569):1195–1202.

Keeling, M. J. and Grenfell, B. T. (1997). Disease extinction and community size: Modeling the persistence of measles. *Science*, 275(5296):65–67.

Keeling, M. J. and Grenfell, B. T. (1998). Effect of variability in infection period on the persistence and spatial spread of infectious diseases. *Mathematical Biosciences*, 147(2):207–226.

Keeling, M. J., Rand, D. A., and Morris, A. J. (1997). Correlation models for childhood epidemics. *Proceedings of the Royal Society of London, Series B, Biological Sciences*, 264(1385):1149–1156.

Keeling, M. J. and Rohani, P. (2002). Estimating spatial coupling in epidemiological systems: A mechanistic approach. *Ecology Letters*, 5(1):20–29.

Keeling, M. J. and Rohani, P. (2007). *Modeling Infectious Diseases in Humans and Animals*. Princeton University Press, Princeton, NJ.

Keeling, M. J., Woolhouse, M. E. J., May, R. M., Davies, G., and Grenfell, B. T. (2003). Modelling vaccination strategies against foot-and-mouth disease. *Nature*, 421(6919):136–142.

Keeling, M. J., Woolhouse, M. E. J., Shaw, D. J., Matthews, L., Chase-Topping, M., Haydon, D. T., Cornell, S. J., Kappey, J., Wilesmith, J., and Grenfell, B. T. (2001). Dynamics of the 2001 UK foot and mouth epidemic: Stochastic dispersal in a heterogeneous landscape. *Science*, 294(5543):813–817.

Kermack, W. O. and McKendrick, A. G. (1927). A contribution to the mathematical theory of epidemics. *Proceedings of the Royal Society of London, Series A, Mathematical and Physical Sciences*, 115:700–721.

Kirchoff, G. (1847). Über die auflösung der gleichungen, auf welche man bei der untersuchung der linearen Vertheilung galvanischer ströme geführt wird. *Annalen der Physik*, 148:497–508.

Kitching, R. P., Hutber, A. M., and Thrusfield, M. V. (2005). A review of foot-and-mouth disease with special consideration for the clinical and epidemiological factors relevant to predictive modelling of the disease. *Veterinary Journal*, 169(2):197–209.

Kitching, R. P., Taylor, N. M., and Thrusfield, M. V. (2007). Vaccination strategies for foot-and-mouth disease. *Nature*, 445:E12.

Kitching, R. P., Thrusfield, M. V., and Taylor, N. M. (2006). Use and abuse of mathematical models: An illustration from the 2001 foot and mouth epidemic in the United Kingdom. *Revue Scientifique et Technique de L'Office International des Épizooties*, 25(1):293–311.

Kitron, U. and Kazmierczak, J. J. (1997). Spatial analysis of the distribution of Lyme disease in Wisconsin. *American Journal of Epidemiology*, 145(6):558–566.

Klauber, M. R. and Angulo, J. J. (1976). Variola minor in Braganca Paulista county, 1956. Attack rates in various population units of the two schools including most students with the disease. *American Journal of Epidemiology*, 103(1):112–125.

Klemm, K. and Eguiluz, V. M. (2002). Growing scale-free networks with small-world behavior. *Physical Review E*, 65(5 Pt 2):057102.

Kloeden, P. E. and Platen, E. (1999). *Numerical Solution of Stochastic Differential Equations*. Applications of Mathematics 23. Springer, New York.

Klovdahl, A. S. (1985). Social networks and the spread of infectious diseases: The AIDS example. *Social Science and Medicine*, 21:1203–1216.

Knox, E. G. (1980). Strategy for rubella vaccination. *International Journal of Epidemiology*, 9:13–23.

Kolmogoroff, A. N., Petrovsky, I. G., and Piscounoff, N. S. (1937). Etude de l'equation de la diffusion avec croissance de la quantite de matiere et son application a un probleme biologique. *Bulletin de l'Universite a Moscou (ser intern)*, A1:1–25.

Koopman, J. S., Chick, S. E., Riolo, C. S., Adams, A. L., Wilson, M. L., and Becker, M. P. (2000). Modeling contact networks and infection transmission in geographic and social space using GERMS. *Sexually Transmitted Diseases*, 27(10):617–626.

Kretzschmar, M. (2000). Sexual network structure and sexually transmitted disease prevention: A modeling perspective. *Sexually Transmitted Diseases*, 27(10):627–635.

Kretzschmar, M. (2002). Mathematical epidemiology of *Chlamydia trachomatis* infections. *Netherlands Journal of Medicine*, 60(7 Suppl):35–43.

Kretzschmar, M. and Morris, M. (1996). Measures of concurrency in networks and the spread of infectious disease. *Mathematical Biosciences*, 133(2):165–195.

Kretzschmar, M., Reinking, D. P., Brouwers, H., van Zessen, G., and Jager, J. C. (1994). Network models: From paradigm to mathematical tool. In Kaplan, E. H. and Brandeau, M. L., editors, *Modeling the AIDS Epidemic: Planning, Policy, and Prediction*, pages 561–583. Raven Press, New York.

Kretzschmar, M., van Duynhoven, Y. T., and Severijnen, A. J. (1996). Modeling prevention strategies for gonorrhea and chlamydia using stochastic network simulations. *American Journal of Epidemiology*, 144(3):306–317.

Kulldorff, M. (1998). Statistical methods for spatial epidemiology: Tests for randomness. In Gatrell, A. C. and Löytönen, M., editors, *GIS and Health*, pages 49–62. Taylor and Francis, Philadelphia.

Kulldorff, M. and Nagarwalla, N. (1995). Spatial disease clusters: Detection and inference. *Statistics in Medicine*, 14(8):799–810.

Kuperman, M. and Abramson, G. (2001). Small world effect in an epidemiological model. *Physical Review Letters*, 86:2909–2912.

Kurtz, T. G. (1970). Solutions of ordinary differential equations as limits of pure jump Markov processes. *Journal of Applied Probability*, 7:49–58.

Kurtz, T. G. (1971). Limit theorems for sequences of jump Markov processes approximating ordinary differential equations. *Journal of*

Applied Probability, 8:344–356.

Kuulasmaa, K. (1982). The spatial general epidemic and locally dependent random graphs. *Journal of Applied Probability*, 19:745–758.

Lam, N. S. N., Fan, M., and Liu, K. B. (1996). Spatial-temporal spread of the AIDS epidemic, 1982-1990: A correlogram analysis of four regions of the United States. *Geographical Analysis*, 28(2):93–107.

Leinhardt, S., editor (1977). *Social Networks: A Developing Paradigm*. Academic Press, New York.

Lewis, M. A. (2000). Spread rate for a nonlinear stochastic invasion. *Journal of Mathematical Biology*, 41:430–454.

Lewis, M. A. and Pacala, S. (2000). Modeling and analysis of stochastic invasion processes. *Journal of Mathematical Biology*, 41(5):387–429.

Li, W. and Cai, X. (2004). Statistical analysis of airport network of China. *Physical Review E*, 69:046106.

Lidwell, O. M. and Williams, R. E. (1961). The epidemiology of the common cold. *Journal of Hygiene–Cambridge*, 59:309–319.

Liljeros, F., Edling, C. R., Amaral, L. A., Stanley, H. E., and Aberg, Y. (2001). The web of human sexual contacts. *Nature*, 411(6840):907–908.

Liljeros, F., Edling, C. R., Stanley, H. E., Aberg, Y., and Amaral, L. A. (2003). Sexual contacts and epidemic thresholds: Reply. *Nature*, 423:606.

Lipsitch, M., Cohen, T., Cooper, B., Robins, J. M., Ma, S., James, L., Gopalakrishna, G., Chew, S. K., Tan, C. C., Samore, M. H., Fisman, D., and Murray, M. (2003). Transmission dynamics and control of severe acute respiratory syndrome. *Science*, 300:1966–1970.

Lloyd, A. L. (2001a). Destabilization of epidemic models with the inclusion of realistic distributions of infectious periods. *Proceedings of the Royal Society of London, Series B, Biological Sciences*, 268(1470):985–993.

Lloyd, A. L. (2001b). Realistic distributions of infectious periods in epidemic models: Changing patterns of persistence and dynamics. *Theoretical Population Biology*, 60(1):59–71.

Lloyd, A. L. (2004). Estimating variability in models for recurrent epidemics: Assessing the use of moment closure techniques. *Theoretical Population Biology*, 65(1):49–65.

Lloyd, A. L. and Jansen, V. A. A. (2004). Spatiotemporal dynamics of epidemics: Synchrony in metapopulation models. *Mathematical Biosciences*, 188:1–16.

Lloyd, A. L. and May, R. M. (1996). Spatial heterogeneity in epidemic models. *Journal of Theoretical Biology*, 179(1):1–11.

Lloyd, A. L. and May, R. M. (2001). How viruses spread among computers and people. *Science*, 292(5520):1316–1317.

Lloyd-Smith, J. O., Galvani, A. P., and Getz, W. M. (2003). Controlling transmission of severe acute respiratory syndrome within a community and its hospital. *Proceedings of the Royal Society of London, Series B, Biological Sciences*, 270:1979–1989.

London, W. P. and Yorke, J. A. (1973). Recurrent outbreaks of measles, chickenpox, and mumps, I: Seasonal variation in contact rates. *American Journal of Epidemiology*, 98:453–468.

Longini, Jr., I. M. (1988). A mathematical model for predicting the geographic spread of new infectious agents. *Mathematical Biosciences*, 90(1-2):367–383.

Longini, Jr., I. M., Clark, W. S., Byers, R. H., Ward, J. W., Darrow, W. W., Lemp, G. F., and Hethcote, H. W. (1989). Statistical analysis of the stages of HIV infection using a Markov model. *Statistics in Medicine*, 8(7):831–843.

Longini, Jr., I. M., Fine, P. E., and Thacker, S. B. (1986). Predicting the global spread of new infectious agents. *American Journal of Epidemiology*, 123(3):383–391.

Longini, Jr., I. M., Nizam, A., Xu, S., Ungchusak, K., Hanshaoworakul, W., Cummings, D. A. T., and Halloran, M. (2005). Containing pandemic influenza at the source. *Science*, 309(5737):1083–1087.

Löytönen, M. (1991). The spatial diffusion of human immunodeficiency virus type 1 in Finland, 1982-1997. *Annals of the Association of American Geographers*, 81:127–151.

Löytönen, M. (1994). Growth models and the HIV epidemic in Finland. *Social Science and Medicine*, 38(1):179–185.

Löytönen, M. and Arbona, S. I. (1996). Forecasting the AIDS epidemic in Puerto Rico. *Social Science and Medicine*, 42(7):997–1010.

Löytönen, M. and Maasilta, P. (1997). Forecasting the HIV epidemic in Finland by using functional small area units. *GeoJournal*, 41(3):215–222.

Luce, R. D. (1950). Connectivity and generalized cliques in sociometric group structure. *Psychometrika*, 15:169–190.

Macdonald, G. (1952). The analysis of equilibrium in malaria. *Tropical Diseases Bulletin*, 49:813–829.

Malice, M. P. and Kryscio, R. J. (1989). On the role of variable incubation periods in simple epidemic models. *IMA Journal of Mathematics Applied in Medicine and Biology*, 6(4):233–242.

Markel, H. (1997). *QUARANTINE! East European Jewish Immigrants and the New York City Epidemics of 1892*. The Johns Hopkins University Press, Baltimore.

Marshall, R. J. (1991). A review of methods for the statistical analysis of spatial patterns of disease. *Journal of the Royal Statistical Society, Series A, Statistics in Society*, 154(3):421–441.

Matinovic, J. (1969). A short history of quarantine. *University of Michigan Medical Journal*, 35:224–228.

Matsuda, M., Ogita, N., Sasaki, A., and Sato, K. (1992). Statistical mechanisms of population. *Progress in Theoretical Physics*, 88:1035–1049.

Matthews, L., Haydon, D. T., Shaw, D. J., Chase-Topping, M. E., Keeling, M. J., and Woolhouse, M. E. (2003). Neighbourhood control policies and the spread of infectious diseases. *Proceedings of the Royal Society of London, Series B, Biological Sciences*, 270(1525):1659–1666.

May, R. M. and Anderson, R. M. (1984). Spatial heterogeneity and the design of immunization programs. *Mathematical Biosciences*, 72:83–111.

May, R. M. and Anderson, R. M. (1988). The transmission dynamics of human immunodeficiency virus (HIV). *Philosophical Transactions of the Royal Society of London, Series B, Biological Sciences*, 321:565–607.

May, R. M. and Lloyd, A. L. (2001). Infection dynamics on scale-free networks. *Physical Review E*, 64:066112.

McCallum, H., Barlow, N., and Hone, J. (2001). How should pathogen transmission be modelled? *Trends in Ecology and Evolution*, 16:295–300.

McKee Jr., K. T., Shields, T. M., Jenkins, P. R., Zenilman, J. M., and Glass, G. E. (2000). Application of a geographic information system to the tracking and control of an outbreak of shigellosis. *Clinical Infectious Diseases*, 31(3):728–733.

Meade, M. S. and Earickson, R. J. (2000). *Medical Geography*. Guilford Press, New York.

Metz, J. A. J. and Diekmann, O. (1986). *The Dynamics of Physio-*

logically Structured Populations. Lecture Notes in Biomathematics 68. Springer-Verlag, New York.

Metz, J. A. J., Mollison, D., and van den Bosch, F. (2000). The dynamics of invasion waves. In Dieckmann, U., Law, R., and Metz, J. A. J., editors, *The Geometry of Ecological Interactions: Simplifying Spatial Complexity.* Cambridge University Press, Cambridge.

Meyers, L. A., Pourbohloul, B., Newman, M. E., Skowronski, D. M., and Brunham, R. C. (2005). Network theory and SARS: Predicting outbreak diversity. *Journal of Theoretical Biology,* 232(1):71–81.

Mielke, J. H., Jorde, L. B., Trapp, P. G., Anderton, D. L., Pitkänen, K., and Eriksson, A. W. (1984). Historical epidemiology of smallpox in Åland, Finland: 1751-1890. *Demography,* 24:271–295.

Milgram, S. (1967). The small world problem. *Psychology Today,* 2:60–67.

Miller, J. M. (1993). Vignette of medical history: Lazaretto Point. *Maryland Medical Journal,* 42:1123–1125.

Mollison, D. (1977). Spatial contact models for ecological and epidemic spread. *Journal of the Royal Statistical Society, Series B, Statistical Methodology,* 39:283–326.

Mollison, D. (1991). Dependence of epidemic and population velocities on basic parameters. *Mathematical Biosciences,* 107:255–287.

Mollison, D. and Kuulasmaa, K. (1985). Spatial epidemic models: Theory and simulations. In Bacon, P., editor, *Population Dynamics of Rabies in Wildlife,* pages 291–309. Academic Press, London.

Moncayo, A. C., Edman, J. D., and Finn, J. T. (2000). Application of geographic information technology in determining risk of eastern equine encephalomyelitis virus transmission. *Journal of the American Mosquito Control Association,* 16(1):28–35.

Monto, A. S. (1968). A community study of respiratory infections in the tropics, 3: Introduction and transmission of infections within families. *American Journal of Epidemiology,* 88(1):69–79.

Moore, D. A. and Carpenter, T. E. (1999). Spatial analytical methods and geographic information systems: Use in health research and epidemiology. *Epidemiologic Reviews,* 21(2):143–161.

Moreno, J. L. (1934). *Who Shall Survive?: A New Approach to the Problem of Human Interrelations.* Nervous and Mental Disease Publishing Company, Washington, DC.

Morris, M. (1993). Epidemiology and social networks: Modeling structured diffusion. *Sociological Methods and Research,* 22(1):99–126.

Morris, M., editor (2004a). *Network Epidemiology: A Handbook for Survey Design and Data Collection*. Oxford University Press, Oxford.

Morris, M. (2004b). Overview of network survey designs. In Morris, M., editor, *Network Epidemiology: A Handbook for Survey Design and Data Collection*, pages 8–21. Oxford University Press, Oxford.

Morris, M. and Kretzschmar, M. (1995). Concurrent partnerships and transmission dynamics in networks. *Social Networks*, 17(3-4):299–318.

Morris, M. and Kretzschmar, M. (1997). Concurrent partnerships and the spread of HIV. *AIDS*, 11(5):641–648.

Morris, M., Podhisita, C., Wawer, M. J., and Handcock, M. S. (1996). Bridge populations in the spread of HIV/AIDS in Thailand. *AIDS*, 10(11):1265–1271.

Morris, R. S., Wilesmith, J. W., Stern, M. W., Sanson, R. L., and Stevenson, M. A. (2001). Predictive spatial modelling of alternative control strategies for the foot-and-mouth disease epidemic in Great Britain, 2001. *Veterinary Record*, 149(5):137–144.

Morrison, A. C., Getis, A., Santiago, M., Rigau-Perez, J. G., and Reiter, P. (1998). Exploratory space-time analysis of reported dengue cases during an outbreak in Florida, Puerto Rico, 1991-1992. *American Journal of Tropical Medicine and Hygiene*, 58(3):287–298.

Mort, M., Convery, I., Baxter, J., and Bailey, C. (2005). Psychosocial effects of the 2001 UK foot and mouth disease epidemic in a rural population: Qualitative diary based study. *British Medical Journal*, 331:1234–1238.

Moutou, F. (2002). Epidemiological basis useful for the control of foot-and-mouth disease. *Comparative Immunology, Microbiology, and Infectious Diseases*, 25(5-6):321–330.

Moutou, F. and Durand, B. (1994). Modelling the spread of foot-and-mouth disease virus. *Veterinary Research*, 25(2-3):279–285.

Murray, G. D. and Cliff, A. D. (1977). A stochastic model for measles epidemics in a multi-region setting. *Transactions of the Institute of British Geographers*, 2:158–174.

Murray, J. D. (1987). Modeling the spread of rabies. *American Scientist*, 75:280–284.

Murray, J. D. (1989). *Mathematical Biology*. Springer-Verlag, New York.

Murray, J. D., Stanley, E. A., and Brown, D. L. (1986). On the spatial spread of rabies among foxes. *Proceedings of the Royal Society of London, Series B, Biological Sciences*, 229(1255):111–150.

Musto, D. F. (1988). Quarantine and the problem of AIDS. In Fee, E. and Fox, D. M., editors, *AIDS: The Burdens of History*, pages 67–84. University of California Press, Los Angeles.

Nåsell, I. (1999). On the time to extinction in recurrent epidemics. *Journal of the Royal Statistical Society, Series B, Statistical Methodology*, 61:309–330.

Newman, M. E. J. (2002a). Assortative mixing in networks. *Physical Review Letters*, 89:208701.

Newman, M. E. J. (2002b). Spread of epidemic diseases on networks. *Physical Review E*, 66:016128.

Newman, M. E. J. (2003a). Ego-centered networks and the ripple effect. *Social Networks*, 25:83–95.

Newman, M. E. J. (2003b). Mixing patterns in networks. *Physical Review E*, 67:026126.

Newman, M. E. J. (2003c). Properties of highly clustered networks. *Physical Review E*, 68:026121.

Newman, M. E. J. (2003d). The structure and function of complex networks. *SIAM Review*, 45:167–256.

Nielen, M., Jalvingh, A. W., Meuwissen, M. P., Horst, S. H., and Dijkhuizen, A. A. (1999). Spatial and stochastic simulation to evaluate the impact of events and control measures on the 1997-1998 classical swine fever epidemic in the Netherlands, II: Comparison of control strategies. *Preventive Veterinary Medicine*, 42(3-4):297–317.

Nisbet, R. M. and Gurney, W. S. C. (1982). *Modelling Fluctuating Populations*. Wiley, New York.

Nisbet, R. M. and Gurney, W. S. C. (1986). The formulation of age-structured models. In Hallam, T. G. and Levin, S. A., editors, *Mathematical Ecology: An Introduction*, Biomathematics 17. Springer-Verlag, New York.

Noble, J. V. (1974). Geographic and temporal development of plagues. *Nature*, 250(5469):726–729.

Nold, A. (1980). Heterogeneity in disease-transmission modeling. *Mathematical Biosciences*, 52:227–240.

North, M. J., Collier, N. T., and Vos, J. R. (2006). Experiences creating three implementations of the Repast agent modeling toolkit. *ACM Transactions on Modeling and Computer Simulation*, 16:1–

25.

Nowak, M. A., Lloyd, A. L., Vasquez, G. M., Wiltrout, T. A., Wahl, L. M., Bischofberger, N., Williams, J., Kinter, A., Fauci, A. S., Hirsch, V. M., and Lifson, J. D. (1997). Viral dynamics of primary viremia and antiretroviral therapy in simian immunodeficiency virus infection. *Journal of Virology*, 71(10):7518–7525.

Øksendal, B. K. (1998). *Stochastic Differential Equations: An Introduction with Applications*. Springer, New York, 5th edition.

Olff, M., Koeter, M. W. J., Van Haaften, E. H., Kersten, P. H., and Gersons, B. P. R. (2005). Impact of a foot and mouth disease crisis on post-traumatic stress symptoms in farmers. *British Journal of Psychiatry*, 186:165–166.

Olsen, L. F., Truty, G. L., and Schaffer, W. M. (1988). Oscillations and chaos in epidemics: A nonlinear dynamic study of six childhood diseases in Copenhagen, Denmark. *Theoretical Population Biology*, 33(3):344–370.

Olson, D. R., Simonsen, L., Edelson, P. J., and Morse, S. S. (2005). Epidemiological evidence of an early wave of the 1918 influenza pandemic in New York City. *Proceedings of the National Academy of Sciences of the United States of America*, 102(31):11059–11063.

Ooi, P. L., Lim, S., and Chew, S. K. (2005). Use of quarantine in the control of SARS in Singapore. *American Journal of Infection Control*, 33(5):252–257.

Oxford, J. S. (2001). The so-called Great Spanish Influenza Pandemic of 1918 may have originated in France in 1916. *Philosophical Transactions of the Royal Society of London*, B, 356:1857–1859.

Oxford, J. S., Sefton, A., Jackson, R., Innes, W., Daniels, R. S., and Johnson, N. P. A. S. (2002). World War I may have allowed the emergence of "Spanish" influenza. *The Lancet Infectious Diseases*, 2:111–114.

Palese, P. (1993). Evolution of influenza and RNA viruses. In Morse, S. J., editor, *Emerging Viruses*, pages 226–233. Oxford University Press, Oxford.

Pang, X., Zhu, Z., Xu, F., Guo, J., Gong, X., Liu, D., Liu, Z., Chin, D. P., and Felkin, D. R. (2003). Evaluation of control measures implemented in the Severe Acute Respiratory Syndrome outbreak in Beijing, 2003. *Journal of the American Medical Association*, 290(24):3215–3221.

Pantaleo, G., Graziosi, C., and Fauci, A. S. (1993). New concepts in the immunopathogenesis of human immunodeficiency virus infection. *New England Journal of Medicine*, 328(5):327–335.

Panum, P. L. (1847). Iagttagelser anstillede under maeslinge-epidermien paa Faeroerne i Aaret 1846. *Bibliothek for Laeger*, 1:270–344.

Panum, P. L. (1939). Observations made during the epidemic of measles in the Faeroe Islands in the year 1846. *Medical Classics*, 3:803–886.

Pastor-Satorras, R. and Vespignani, A. (2001a). Epidemic dynamics and endemic states in complex networks. *Physical Review E*, 63:066117.

Pastor-Satorras, R. and Vespignani, A. (2001b). Epidemic spreading in scale-free networks. *Physical Review Letters*, 86(14):3200–3203.

Pastor-Satorras, R. and Vespignani, A. (2002). Immunization of complex networks. *Physical Review E*, 65:036104.

Peiris, J. S. M., Yuen, K. Y., Osterhaus, A. D. M. E., and Stohr, K. (2003). Current concepts: The severe acute respiratory syndrome. *The New England Journal of Medicine*, 349(25):2431–2441.

Peterman, T. A., Stoneburner, R. L., Allen, J. R., Jaffe, H. W., and Curran, J. W. (1988). Risk of human immunodeficiency virus transmission from heterosexual adults with transfusion-associated infections. *Journal of the American Medical Association*, 259:55–58.

Pfeiffer, D. U. and Hugh-Jones, M. (2002). Geographical information systems as a tool in epidemiological assessment and wildlife disease management. *Revue Scientifique et Technique de L'Office International des Épizooties*, 21(1):91–102.

Pool, I. and Kochen, M. (1978). Contacts and influence. *Social Networks*, 1:1–48.

Post, W. M., DeAngelis, D. L., and Travis, C. C. (1983). Endemic disease in environments with spatially heterogeneous host populations. *Mathematical Biosciences*, 63:289–302.

Potter, C. W. (2001). A history of influenza. *Journal of Applied Microbiology*, 91:572–579.

Potterat, J. J., Woodhouse, D. E., Muth, S. Q., Rothenberg, R. B., Darrow, W. W., Klovdahl, A. S., and Muth, J. B. (2004). Network dynamism: History and lessons of the Colorado Springs study. In Morris, M., editor, *Network Epidemiology: A Handbook for Survey Design and Data Collection*, pages 87–114. Oxford University Press, Oxford.

Press, W. H., Teukolsky, S. A., Vetterling, W. T., and Flannery, B. P. (1996). *Numerical Recipes in FORTRAN: The Art of Scientific*

Computing. Cambridge University Press, Cambridge, 2nd edition.

Rand, D. (1999). Correlation equations and pair approximations for spatial ecologies. In McGlade, E., editor, *Advanced Ecological Theory: Principles and Applications*, pages 100–142. Blackwell Science, Oxford.

Rapoport, A. (1957). Contribution to the theory of random and biased nets. *Bulletin of Mathematical Biophysics*, 19:257–277.

Rapoport, A. and Horvath, W. J. (1961). A study of a large sociogram. *Behavioral Sciences*, 6:279–291.

Rass, L. and Radcliffe, J. (2003). *Spatial Deterministic Epidemics*. American Mathematical Society, Providence, RI.

Reid, A. H., Taubenberger, J. K., and Fanning, T. G. (2004). Evidence of an absence: The genetic origins of the 1918 pandemic influenza virus. *Nature Reviews Microbiology*, 2:909–914.

Renshaw, E. (1991). *Modelling Biological Populations in Space and Time*. Cambridge Studies in Mathematical Biology 11. Cambridge University Press, Cambridge.

Rhodes, C. J. and Anderson, R. M. (1996). A scaling analysis of measles epidemics in a small population. *Philosophical Transactions of the Royal Society of London, Series B, Biological Sciences*, 351:1679–1688.

Riley, S., Fraser, C., Donnelly, C. A., Ghani, A. C., Abu-Raddad, L. J., Hedley, A. J., Leung, G. M., Ho, L.-M., Lam, T.-H., Thach, T. Q., Chau, P., Chan, K.-P., Lo, S.-V., Leung, P.-Y., Tsang, T., Ho, W., Lee, K.-H., Lau, E. M. C., Ferguson, N. M., and Anderson, R. M. (2003). Transmission dynamics of the etiological agent of SARS in Hong Kong: Impact of public health interventions. *Science*, 300:1961–1966.

Rivas, A. L., Tennenbaum, S. E., Aparicio, J. P., Hoogesteijn, A. L., Mohammed, H. O., Castillo-Chavez, C., and Schwager, S. J. (2003). Critical response time (time available to implement effective measures for epidemic control): Model building and evaluation. *Canadian Journal of Veterinary Research*, 67(4):307–311.

Roberts, F. S. (1976). *Discrete Mathematical Models with Applications to Social, Biological, and Environmental Problems*. Prentice-Hall, Englewood Cliffs, NJ.

Roberts, F. S. (1979). Graph theory and the social sciences. In Wilson, R. J. and Beineke, L. W., editors, *Applications of Graph Theory*, pages 255–291. Academic Press, New York.

Robinson, T. P. (2000). Spatial statistics and geographical information systems in epidemiology and public health. *Advances in Parasitology*, 47:81–128.

Roethlisberger, F. J. and Dickson, W. J. (1939). *Management and the Worker*. Harvard University Press, Cambridge, MA.

Rohani, P., Earn, D. J., Finkenstädt, B. F., and Grenfell, B. T. (1998). Population dynamic interference among childhood diseases. *Proceedings of the Royal Society of London, Series B, Biological Sciences*, 265(1410):2033–2041.

Rohani, P., Earn, D. J., and Grenfell, B. T. (1999). Opposite patterns of synchrony in sympatric disease metapopulations. *Science*, 286(5441):968–971.

Rohani, P., Green, C. J., Mantilla-Beniers, N. B., and Grenfell, B. T. (2003). Ecological interference between fatal diseases. *Nature*, 422(6934):885–888.

Rohani, P., Keeling, M. J., and Grenfell, B. T. (2002). The interplay between determinism and stochasticity in childhood diseases. *American Naturalist*, 159(5):469–481.

Rozenfeld, A. F., Cohen, R., Ben-Avraham, D., and Havlin, S. (2002). Scale-free networks on lattices. *Physical Review Letters*, 89(21):218701.

Rushton, G. (1998). Improving the geographic basis of health surveillance using GIS. In Gatrell, A. C. and Löytönen, M., editors, *GIS and Health*, pages 63–79. Taylor and Francis, Philadelphia.

Rushton, S. P. and Mautner, A. (1955). The deterministic model of a simple epidemic for more than one community. *Biometrika*, 42:126–132.

Rvachev, L. A. and Longini, Jr., I. M. (1985). A mathematical model for the global spread of influenza. *Mathematical Biosciences*, 75(1):1–22.

Salt, J. S., Barnett, P. V., Dani, P., and Williams, L. (1998). Emergency vaccination of pigs against foot-and-mouth disease: Protection against disease and reduction in contact transmission. *Vaccine*, 16(7):746–754.

Sanson, R. L., Morris, R. S., and Stern, M. W. (1999). EpiMAN-FMD: A decision support system for managing epidemics of vesicular disease. *Revue Scientifique et Technique de L'Office International des Épizooties*, 18(3):593–605.

Sartwell, P. E. (1950). The distribution of incubation periods of infectious disease. *American Journal of Hygiene*, 51:310–318.

Sartwell, P. E. (1966). The incubation period and dynamics of infectious disease. *American Journal of Epidemiology*, 83:204–216.

Sato, K., Matsuda, H., and Sasaki, A. (1994). Pathogen invasion and host extinction in lattice structured populations. *Journal of Mathematical Biology*, 32(3):251–268.

Sattenspiel, L. (1987a). Epidemics in nonrandomly mixing populations: A simulation. *American Journal of Physical Anthropology*, 73(2):251–265.

Sattenspiel, L. (1987b). Population structure and the spread of disease. *Human Biology*, 59(3):411–438.

Sattenspiel, L. and Dietz, K. (1995). A structured epidemic model incorporating geographic mobility among regions. *Mathematical Biosciences*, 128(1-2):71–91.

Sattenspiel, L. and Herring, D. A. (1998). Structured epidemic models and the spread of influenza in the central Canadian subarctic. *Human Biology*, 70(1):91–115.

Sattenspiel, L. and Herring, D. A. (2003). Simulating the effect of quarantine on the spread of the 1918-19 flu in central Canada. *Bulletin of Mathematical Biology*, 65(1):1–26.

Sattenspiel, L., Mobarry, A., and Herring, D. A. (2000). Modeling the influence of settlement structure on the spread of influenza among communities. *American Journal of Human Biology*, 12(6):736–748.

Sattenspiel, L. and Simon, C. (1988). The spread and persistence of infectious diseases in structured populations. *Mathematical Biosciences*, 90:341–366.

Schaffer, W. M. (1985). Can nonlinear dynamics elucidate mechanisms in ecology and epidemiology? *IMA Journal of Mathematics Applied in Medicine and Biology*, 2(4):221–252.

Schaffer, W. M. and Kot, M. (1985). Nearly one dimensional dynamics in an epidemic. *Journal of Theoretical Biology*, 112:403–427.

Schenzle, D. (1984). An age-structured model of pre- and post-vaccination measles transmission. *IMA Journal of Mathematics Applied in Medicine and Biology*, 1(2):169–191.

Schenzle, D. and Dietz, K. (1987). Critical population sizes for endemic virus transmission. In Fricke, W. and Hinz, E., editors, *Räumliche Persistenz und Diffusion von Krankheiten*, pages 31–42. Heidelberger Geographische Arbeiten, Heidelberg.

Schneeberger, A., Mercer, C. H., Gregson, S. A. J., Ferguson, N. M., Nyamukapa, C. A., Anderson, R. M., Johnson, A. M., and Garnett, G. P. (2004). Scale-free networks and sexually transmitted diseases — a description of observed patterns of sexual contacts in Britain and Zimbabwe. *Sexually Transmitted Diseases*, 31(6):380–387.

Scholtissek, C. (1994). Source for influenza pandemics. *European Journal of Epidemiology*, 10(4):455–458.

Schrag, S. J., Brooks, J. T., Van Beneden, C., Parashar, U. D., Griffin, P. M., Anderson, L. J., Bellini, W. J., Benson, R. F., Erdman, D. D., Klimov, A., Ksiazek, T. G., Peret, T. C. T., Talkington, D. F., Thacker, W. L., Tondella, M. L., Sampson, J. S., Hightower, A. W., Nordenberg, D. F., Plikaytis, B. D., Khan, A. S., Rosenstein, N. E., Treadwell, T. A., Whitney, C. G., Fiore, A. E., Durant, T. M., Perz, J. F., Wasley, A., Feikin, D., Herndon, J. L., Bower, W. A., Kilbourn, B. W., Levy, D. A., Coronado, V. G., Buffington, J., Dykewicz, C. A., Khabbaz, R. F., and Chamberland, M. E. (2004). SARS surveillance during emergency public health response, United States, March-July 2003. *Emerging Infectious Diseases*, 10(2):185–194.

Schwartz, I. B. (1992). Small amplitude, long period outbreaks in seasonally driven epidemics. *Journal of Mathematical Biology*, 30(5):473–491.

Simonsen, L., Clarke, M. J., Schonberger, L. B., Arden, N. H., Cox, N. J., and Fukuda, K. (1998). Pandemic versus epidemic influenza mortality: A pattern of changing age distribution. *Journal of Infectious Diseases*, 178(1):53–60.

Smallman-Raynor, M. R. and Cliff, A. D. (1991). Civil war and the spread of AIDS in Central Africa. *Epidemiology and Infection*, 107(1):69–80.

Smallman-Raynor, M. R. and Cliff, A. D. (1998a). *Deciphering Global Epidemics: Analytical Approaches to the Disease Records of World Cities, 1888-1912*. Cambridge University Press, Cambridge.

Smallman-Raynor, M. R. and Cliff, A. D. (1998b). The Philippines insurrection and the 1902-4 cholera epidemic, part I: Epidemiological diffusion processes in war. *Journal of Historical Geography*, 24(1):69–89.

Smallman-Raynor, M. R. and Cliff, A. D. (1998c). The Philippines insurrection and the 1902-4 cholera epidemic, part II: Diffusion patterns in war and peace. *Journal of Historical Geography*, 24(2):188–210.

Smallman-Raynor, M. R. and Cliff, A. D. (2001a). Epidemic diffusion processes in a system of US military camps: Transfer diffusion and the spread of typhoid fever in the Spanish-American War, 1898. *Annals of the Association of American Geographers*, 91(1):71–91.

Smallman-Raynor, M. R. and Cliff, A. D. (2001b). Epidemiological spaces: The use of multidimensional scaling to identify cholera diffusion processes in wake of the Philippines insurrection, 1899-1902. *Transactions of the Institute of British Geographers*, 26(3):288–305.

Smith, D. L., Lucey, B., Waller, L. A., Childs, J. E., and Real, L. A. (2002). Predicting the spatial dynamics of rabies epidemics on heterogeneous landscapes. *Proceedings of the National Academy of Sciences of the United States of America*, 99(6):3668–3672.

Smith, P. and Thomas, R. (2001). Epidemic modelling of HIV/AIDS transfers between eastern and western Europe. *GeoJournal*, 53(4):373–383.

Soper, M. A. (1929). The interpretation of periodicity in disease prevalence. *Journal of the Royal Statistical Society, Series A, Statistics in Society*, 92:34–61.

Sorensen, J. H., Mackay, D. K. J., Jensen, C. O., and Donaldson, A. I. (2000). An integrated model to predict the atmospheric spread of foot-and-mouth disease virus. *Epidemiology and Infection*, 124(3):577–590.

Spencer, F. (1967). Port health services through the ages. *Royal Institute of Public Health and Hygiene Journal*, 30:88–91.

Spicer, C. C. (1979). The mathematical modelling of influenza epidemics. *British Medical Bulletin*, 35(1):23–28.

Stauffer, D. and Aharony, A. (1992). *Introduction to Percolation Theory*. Taylor and Francis, London, 2nd edition.

Stone, L., Olinky, R., and Huppert, A. (2007). Seasonal dynamics of recurrent epidemics. *Nature*, 446:533–536.

Taneyhill, D. E., Dunn, A. M., and Hatcher, M. J. (1999). The Galton-Watson branching process as a quantitative tool in parasitology. *Parasitology Today*, 15(4):159–165.

Taubenberger, J. K. and Morens, D. M. (2006a). 1918 influenza: The mother of all pandemics. *Emerging Infectious Diseases*, 12(1):15–22.

Taubenberger, J. K. and Morens, D. M. (2006b). Influenza revisited. *Emerging Infectious Diseases*, 12(1):1–2.

Taubenberger, J. K., Reid, A. H., and Fanning, T. G. (2000). The 1918 influenza virus: A killer comes into view. *Virology*, 274:241–245.

Thomas, R. W. (2001). Estimated population mixing by country and risk cohort for the HIV/AIDS epidemic in Western Europe. *Journal of Geographic Systems*, 3:283–301.

Thompson, D., Muriel, P., Russell, D., Osborne, P., Bromley, A., Rowland, M., Creigh-Tyte, S., and Brown, C. (2002). Economic costs of the foot and mouth disease outbreak in the United Kingdom in 2001. *Revue Scientifique et Technique de L'Office International des Épizooties*, 21:675–687.

Thompson, W. W., Shay, D. K., Weintraub, E., Brammer, L., Cox, N. J., Anderson, L. J., and Fukuda, K. (2003). Mortality associated with influenza and respiratory syncytial virus in the United States. *Journal of the American Medical Association*, 289(2):179–186.

Thrusfield, M., Mansley, L., Dunlop, P., Taylor, J., and Pawson, A. (2005). The foot-and-mouth disease epidemic in Dumfries and Galloway, 2001, 2: Serosurveillance, and efficiency and effectiveness of control procedures after the national ban on animal movements. *Veterinary Record*, 156:269–278.

Tildesley, M. J., Savill, N. J., Shaw, D. J., Deardon, R., Brooks, S. P., Woolhouse, M. E. J., Grenfell, B. T., and Keeling, M. J. (2006). Optimal reactive vaccination strategy for a foot-and-mouth outbreak in the UK. *Nature*, 440:83–86.

Tildesley, M. J., Savill, N. J., Shaw, D. J., Deardon, R., Brooks, S. P., Woolhouse, M. E. J., Grenfell, B. T., and Keeling, M. J. (2007). Vaccination strategies for foot-and-mouth disease (reply). *Nature*, 445:E12–E13.

Travers, J. and Milgram, S. (1969). An experimental study of the small world problem. *Sociometry*, 32:425–443.

Tsang, T. and Lam, T. H. (2003). SARS: Public health measures in Hong Kong. *Respirology*, 8:S46–S48.

Tuckel, P., Sassler, S., Maisel, R., and Leykam, A. (2006). The diffusion of the influenza pandemic of 1918 in Hartford, Connecticut. *Social Science History*, 30(2):167–196.

Turelli, M. (1977). Random environments and stochastic calculus. *Theoretical Population Biology*, 12(2):140–178.

Turing, A. M. (1952). The chemical basis of morphogenesis. *Philosophical Transactions of the Royal Society of London, Series B, Biological Sciences*, 237:37–72.

van den Bosch, F., Metz, J. A. J., and Diekmann, O. (1990). The velocity of spatial population expansion. *Journal of Mathematical Biology*, 28:529–565.

van den Driessche, P. and Watmough, J. (2002). Reproduction numbers and sub-threshold endemic equilibria for compartmental models of disease transmission. *Mathematical Biosciences*, 180:29–48.

Varia, M., Wilson, S., Sarwal, S., McGeer, A., Gournis, E., Galanis, E., Henry, B., and for the Hospital Outbreak Investigation Team (2003). Investigation of a nosocomial outbreak of severe acute respiratory syndrome (SARS) in Toronto, Canada. *Canadian Medical Association Journal*, 169(4):285–292.

Viboud, C., Bjørnstad, O. N., Smith, D. L., Simonsen, L., Miller, M. A., and Grenfell, B. T. (2006). Synchrony, waves, and spatial hierarchies in the spread of influenza. *Science*, 312:447–451.

Waller, L. A. and Jacquez, G. M. (1995). Disease models implicit in statistical tests of disease clustering. *Epidemiology*, 6(6):584–590.

Waller, L. A. and Lawson, A. B. (1995). The power of focused tests to detect disease clustering. *Statistics in Medicine*, 14(21-22):2291–2308.

Wallinga, J. and Teunis, P. (2004). Different epidemic curves for severe acute respiratory syndrome reveal similar impacts of control measures. *American Journal of Epidemiology*, 160(6):509–516.

Walter, S. D. (2000). Disease mapping: A historical perspective. In Elliott, P., Wakefield, J., Best, N., and Briggs, D., editors, *Spatial Epidemiology: Methods and Applications*, pages 223–239. Oxford University Press, Oxford.

Warren, C. P., Sander, L. M., and Sokolov, I. M. (2002). Geography in a scale-free network model. *Physical Review E*, 66(5 Pt 2):056105.

Wasserman, S. and Faust, K. (1994). *Social Network Analysis: Methods and Applications*. Cambridge University Press, Cambridge.

Watts, D. J., Muhamad, R., Medina, D. C., and Dodds, P. S. (2005). Multiscale, resurgent epidemics in a hierarchical metapopulation model. *Proceedings of the National Academy of Sciences of the United States of America*, 102:11157–11162.

Watts, D. J. and Strogatz, S. H. (1998). Collective dynamics of 'small-world' networks. *Nature*, 393(6684):440–442.

Wawer, M. J., Podhisita, C., Kanungsukkasem, U., Pramualratana, A., and McNamara, R. (1996). Origins and working conditions of female sex workers in urban Thailand: Consequences of social context for HIV transmission. *Social Science and Medicine*, 42(3):453–462.

Webb, G. F., Blaser, M. J., Zhu, H., Ardal, S., and Wu, J. (2004). Critical role of nosocomial transmission in the Toronto SARS outbreak. *Mathematical Biosciences and Engineering*, 1(1):1–13.

Whittle, P. (1955). The outcome of a stochastic epidemic — a note on Bailey's paper. *Biometrika*, 42:116–122.

Whittle, P. (1957). On the use of the normal approximation in the treatment of stochastic processes. *Journal of the Royal Statistical Society, Series B, Statistical Methodology*, 19:268–281.

Williams, J. S. and Rees, P. H. (1994). A simulation of the transmission of HIV and AIDS in regional populations within the United Kingdom. *Transactions of the Institute of British Geographers*, 19(3):311–330.

Wilson, E. B. and Burke, M. H. (1942). The epidemic curve. *Proceedings of the National Academy of Sciences of the United States of America*, 28:361–367.

Wilson, E. B. and Worcester, J. (1945a). Damping of epidemic waves. *Proceedings of the National Academy of Sciences of the United States of America*, 31:294–298.

Wilson, E. B. and Worcester, J. (1945b). The spread of an epidemic. *Proceedings of the National Academy of Sciences of the United States of America*, 31:327–333.

Wingfield, A., Miller, H., and Honhold, N. (2006). FMD control strategies. *Veterinary Record*, 158(20):706–707.

Woolhouse, M. and Donaldson, A. (2001). Managing foot-and-mouth. *Nature*, 410(6828):515–516.

Woolhouse, M. E. (2003). Foot-and-mouth disease in the UK: What should we do next time? *Journal of Applied Microbiology*, 94(Suppl):126S–130S.

Woolhouse, M. E. J., Etard, J.-F., Dietz, K., Ndhlovu, P. D., and Chandiwana, S. K. (1998). Heterogeneities in schistosome transmission dynamics and control. *Parasitology*, 117:475–482.

Xia, Y. C., Bjørnstad, O. N., and Grenfell, B. T. (2004). Measles metapopulation dynamics: A gravity model for epidemiological coupling and dynamics. *American Naturalist*, 164(2):267–281.

Yorke, J. A., Hethcote, H. W., and Nold, A. (1978). Dynamics and control of the transmission of gonorrhea. *Sexually Transmitted Diseases*, 5(2):51–56.

Index

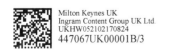
Milton Keynes UK
Ingram Content Group UK Ltd.
UKHW052102170824
447067UK00001B/3

9 780691 121321